T0320561

NEUROPSYCHOLOGICAL REHABILITATION

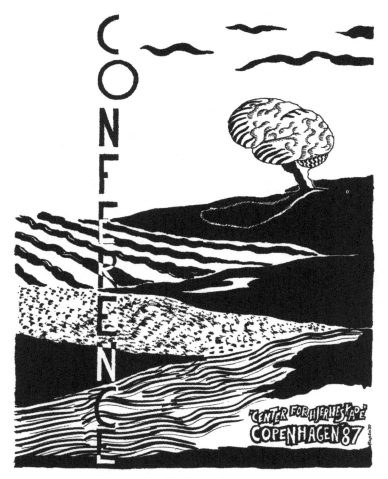

Frontispiece by Hysse Forchhammer

NEUROPSYCHOLOGICAL REHABILITATION

Proceedings of the Conference on Rehabilitation of Brain Damaged People: Current Knowledge and Future Directions, held at Copenhagen, June 15–16, 1987.

Edited by

Anne-Lise Christensen
Barbara P. Uzzell

Kluwer Academic Publishers
Boston   Dordrecht   London

Distributors

for the United States and Canada: Kluwer Academic Publishers, 101 Philip Drive, Assinippi Park, Norwell, MA 02061, USA

for the UK and Ireland: Kluwer Academic Publishers, Falcon House, Queen Square, Lancaster LA1 1RN, UK

for all other countries: Kluwer Academic Publishers, Distribution Centre, Post Office Box 322, 3300 AH Dordrecht, THE NETHERLANDS

Library of Congress Cataloging-in-Publication Data

Conference on Rehabilitation of Brain Damaged People: Current Knowledge and Future Directions (1987 : Copenhagen, Denmark)
  Neuropsychological rehabilitation : proceedings of the Conference on Rehabilitation of Brain Damaged People—Current Knowledge and Future Directions, held at Copenhagen, June 15–16, 1987/edited by Anne-Lise Christensen, Barbara P. Uzzell.
    p. cm.
  Includes index.
  ISBN 0–89838–374–9
  1. Brain damage—Patients—Rehabilitation—Congresses.
I. Christensen, Anne-Lise. II. Uzzell, Barbara P. III. Title.
  [DNLM: 1. Brain Damage, Chronic—rehabilitation—congresses.
2. Brain Injuries—rehabilitation-congresses. 3. Neuropsychology—congresses. WL 354 C748n 1987]
  RC387.5.C68 1987
  617'.481—dc19
  DNLM/DLC   88–5148
  for Library of Congress   CIP

NEUROPSYCHOLOGICAL REHABILITATION: CURRENT KNOWLEDGE AND FUTURE DIRECTIONS

CONTENTS

CONFERENCE	**Rehabilitation af Brain Damaged People:** **Current Knowledge and Future Directions**
PLACE:	Center for Rehabilitation of Brain Damage University of Copenhagen, Amager 88, Njalsgade DK-2300 Copenhagen S., Denmark
TIME:	June 15 - 16, 1987
AIM:	To present and discuss state of the art knowledge within neurophysiology, neurology, neuropharmacology and neuropsychology as they apply to the rehabilitation of brain damaged adults.

PROGRAM

Monday June 15, 1987

MODERATOR:	Erik Strömgren, M.D. Dept. of Psychiatry, University of Aarhus, Aarhus, Denmark.

SPEAKERS:

Donald G. Stein, Ph.D. Office of the Dean of Graduate Studies Rutgers University Newark, New Jersey, U.S.A.	"Experimental approaches to the treatment of brain injuries"
D. Nathan Cope, M.D. The National Rehabilitation Hospital Washington, D.C., U.S.A.	"Neuropharmacology and brain damage"
Lance E. Trexler, Ph.D. Center for Neuropsychological Rehabilitation Indianapolis, Indiana, U.S.A.	"Current research in the rehabili tation of brain damage"
Leonard Diller, Ph.D. Rusk Institute of Rehabilitation Medicine New York University Medical Center New York City, New York, U.S.A.	"Overviews of rehabilitation programs"
Barbara A. Wilson, Ph.D. Department of Rehabilitation Southampton General Hospital Southampton, U.K.	"Future directions in rehabilita- tion of brain damage"
Diana Bistany General Reinsurance Company Stamford, Connecticut, U.S.A.	"The cost – benefits of rehabilitation programs"

PANEL:

Tuesday, June 16, 1987

MODERATOR: Barbara P. Uzzell, Ph.D.
Division of Neurosurgery
Hospital of University of PA.
Philadelphia, PA., U.S.A.

PANEL MEMBERS:

D. Nathan Cope, M.D.
Leonard Diller, Ph.D.
Donald Stein, Ph.D.
Lance Trexler, Ph.D.
Barbara A. Wilson, Ph.D.

DANISH PANEL MEMBERS:

Jens Astrup, M.D.
University of Århus
Århus, Denmark

Fin Biering-Sørensen, M.D.
Dept. of Physical Rehabilitation
Rigshospitalet
Copenhagen, Denmark

Anne-Lise Christensen, Ph.D.
Center for Rehabilitation of Brain
Damage
University of Copenhagen
Copenhagen, Denmark

x

PANEL DISCUSSANTS:

David Ellis, Ph.D.
Brain Injury Center at Plaza Medical
Robert Wood Johnson Medical School at
Camden
Camden, New Jersey, U.S.A.

Arnstein Finset, Ph.D.
Sunnaas Hospital
Nesoddtangen, Norway

Gunilla Øberg, Ph.D.
Dept. of Neurology
Rigshospitalet
Copenhagen, Denmark

Ole Rafaelsen, M.D.
Dept. of Psychiatry
Rigshospitalet
Copenhagen, Denmark

Jarl Risberg, Ph.D.
Dept. of Psychiatry
University of Lund
Lund, Sweden

Ernir Snorrason, M.D.
Dept. of Rehabilitation
Municipal Hospital
Reykjavik, Iceland

Inger Vibeke Thomsen, Ph.D.
Rigshospitalet
Copenhagen, Denmark

Harriet K. Zeiner, Ph.D.
Langley Porter Psychiatric Institute
Dept. of Psychiatry
San Francisco General Hospital
San Francisco, California, U.S.A.

STAFF OF THE CENTER FOR REHABILITATION OF BRAIN DAMAGE:

Anne-Lise Christensen, Director, Neuropsychologist

Inge Albrecht, Clinical Psychologist
Marianne Ewald, Nurse's Aid
Hysse Forchhammer, Psychology Intern
Steen Hartmann, Special Education Teacher
Mette Ishøy, Secretary
Kaj Keiser, Special Education Teacher
Peter Lønberg Madsen, Clinical Psychologist
Finn Malmqvist, Speech Therapist
Grete Mørup, Secretary
Palle Møller Pedersen, Neuropsychologist
Mugge Pinner, Neuropsychologist
Lise Randrup, Neurolinguist
Gitte Rasmussen, Physical Therapist
Nicole K. Rosenberg, Clinical Psychologist

FOREWORD

In early 1985 a grant from the Egmont Foundation
made the establishment of the Center for Rehabilitation
of Brain Damage in Copenhagen possible. This meant the
realization of a plan with which Anne-Lise Christensen
had been occupied for years. Through her work in
psychiatric and neurosurgical wards she had acquired a
deep insight in the problems of the brain damage, and
through visits to the leading centers within the field
of brain damage rehabilitation she had become inti-
mately acquainted with the most modern trends in
research and practice which was insufficiently developed in Denmark. When finally the possibility of
establishing the center came closer, it was obvious
that Anne-Lise Christensen would be the right person to
organize this institution and to become its leader.

Two years later, when the building-up of the
Center had been finished and the work was running
smoothly, it was felt natural to mark this accomplish-
ment by the arrangement of an international conference
on rehabilitation of brain damage. On this occasion, a
number of leading specialists gave lectures on many
different aspects of the topic. This provided great
incentives for those interested in the field in Denmark.

The present volume, containing the lectures from
the conference, can also be regarded as a tribute to
Anne-Lise Christensen and her colleagues, in recognition of their accomplishments within the field of
neuropsychology and rehabilitation of the brain damaged.

Erik Strömgren
Chairman of the Board of Directors
Center for Rehabilitation of Brain Damage

PREFACE

Brain damage has become synonymous with a loss of
skills, while rehabilitation of brain damaged individuals
has become known as a method to restructure lives within
a social context. Until recently, rehabilitation of
brain damaged patients has been limited, confined mainly
to medical treatment and treatment of lost physical
skills. Within the last 10 years changes in rehabilitation have been emerging, as a body of knowledge
from neurophysiology, neurosurgery, neuropharmacology
and neuroimaging with an integration of neuropsychology
into it.

Increasingly, it has become clear that the tragedy
of brain damaged victims is more curtailments or loss of
life transactions, than a loss of physical skills. It is
now apparent that intervention has to be based not only
on integrated knowledge about anatomical location of
lesions, plasticity of the brain, influences of neuro-
biology and neurochemistry, but mainly on integration of
psychological treatment strengthening life transactions.
It is essential that the role of the investigator becomes
that of a collaborator, who reaches out, rather than that
of a test-wielder. This new wave rehabilitation has
influenced the scientific and practical aspects of the
establishment of the Center for Rehabilitation of Brain
Damage at the Psychological Laboratory, University of
Copenhagen, Denmark.

The significance of new wave rehabilitation is the
realization that knowledge needs to be integrated.
Clinically this means that specialists from different
fields talk to one another, recognize the individuality
of the brain damaged victim, develop the most
comprehensive program and address the cost-benefit.

In order to increase awareness of this new kind
of rehabilitation, to stimulate professionals already
engaging in integrated rehabilitation, and to pro-
liferate its growth in Scandinavia, a two day conference was held on June 15 and 16, 1987 in Copenhagen. The conference set the stage for an interaction of various specialists who learned about each
other's viewpoints and research, and then redirected
their beliefs accordingly. Researchers mainly from
the United States, from the United Kingdom, and from
Scandinavia with various backgrounds were invited to
participate. The exchange showed how an integrated
rehabilitation approach unfolds, with one point-of-
view incorporating items from another standpoint.

Because we felt the exchange was timely, important and needed to be available for others not
attending the conference, this book was undertaken.
We hope the reader will share our enthusiasm about
incorporating concepts from other fields into strategies for intervention, will see the cost-benefits
from such an integrated approach to a brain damaged
individual, and will be stimulated by the concepts
and ideas presented in this book.

We want to thank all persons who contributed time
and effort to make this book possible. We especially
want to thank the contributing authors who presented
their points-of-view, and the conference participants
who provoked understanding through their queries and
shared experiences. The final appreciation expressed
is for the generosity of the Egmont Foundation in
making the conference possible and for the financial
support in the initial phases of the Center for
Rehabilitation of Brain Damage.

Anne-Lise Christensen
Barbara P. Uzzell

NEUROPSYCHOLOGICAL REHABILITATION

1

CONTEXTUAL FACTORS IN RECOVERY FROM BRAIN DAMAGE

DONALD G. STEIN

Office of the Dean of the Graduate School and Associate Provost
Rutgers University
Newark, NJ 07102, U.S.A.

I would like to discuss some general concepts of
neuroplasticity and behavior, and the relationship of
this plasticity to the development and organization
of the central nervous system. I will also address
the issue of what neural plasticity means for
understanding rehabilitation from brain injury in its
broadest context. I believe that before one can
examine the question of providing "rehabilitation"
from a neurological or psychological perspective, it
is important to examine some of the physiological
substrates that can account for the different kinds
of 'plasticity' that are manifest in the nervous
system. However, it should be emphasized that just
because the CNS has the <u>potential</u> to function a
certain way, does not necessarily mean that
organismic and environmental conditions will always
be available to operate in the most effective and
adaptive manner. A part of the job of people who are
involved in basic research as well as in clinical
rehabilitation, is to unlock and facilitate the
neuronal mechanisms that underlie both behavioral and
morphological recovery from brain injury.

DEFINING "NEURAL PLASTICITY":

We can begin our discussion by asking the question
of how one defines "neural reality." Is there more
than one way to describe how the brain is organized

Christensen, Anne-Lise and Uzzell, Barbara P. (eds.), *Neuropsychological
Rehabilitation*. Copyright © 1988 Kluwer Academic Publishers. All rights
reserved.

and how it might (or might not) recover from injury? As neuroscientists concerned with CNS functions, we all have our set of truths and our views and beliefs about what constitutes the way in which the nervous system functions. One's perspective on "reality" depends very much on the techniques employed by that discipline to measure phenomena, by what variables are considered worthy of study, and what set of assumptions one has about how the brain works (e.g., see [1]. I suggest that there are different types of 'realities' about nervous system organization that we are only just beginning to understand, and complete understanding may require dramatic shifts in our research paradigms and clinical strategies.

First, though, we need a good definition of "plasticity" as it applies to the central nervous system. We all use the term, but do we have a specific definition? One that I would like to offer is provided by Dr. Bernard Kaplan of Clark University. Referring to the intact organism, Kaplan suggested that "plasticity is the ability to modify organic systems and patterns of behavior." In this particular context, different means can be used to obtain specific, adaptive goals. This definition can apply to the treatment of patients, or in education to achieve a particular objective. With only slight modification, the same definition can also be applied to goal-directed neuronal functions. In this context when we talk about "plasticity," we can ask whether there are varying means that the nervous system uses to achieve very specific functional requirements (e.g., walking, food-getting, problem solving); obviously such means may shift as different demands are made upon the organism. We also can use the term to refer to very widespread <u>individual</u> <u>differences</u> in response to both external and internal milieu. The key to understanding neural plasticity may lie in the study of individual differences; a viewpoint which seems to have fallen from favor.

One aspect of plasticity that I think is important for scientists and especially for rehabilitation practitioners to recognize is that the term cannot be defined in some abstract way. One must refer to the particular means that are used to achieve specific ends. A developmental analysis of plastic phenomena is, in one sense, an analysis of the means that organisms use to accomplish goals. In the final analysis, in the study of CNS plasticity, it might be better to approach the problem from a developmental perspective. Here, I do not mean development to imply the study of child behavior or simple growth; development does not 'reside' in the organism. First, it is a concept that we can apply to examine the kinds of changes that take place as we make different interventions to promote specific goals. Second, we can characterize developmental processes in terms of events that can alter the ability of the nervous system to adapt to various kinds of trauma, disintegration and reorganization that can occur after injury. In this context we are actually examining the capacity of the nervous system to repair itself as well as the events and conditions which might block that repair.

Eugene Gollin (2) defines plasticity as the "possible range of variations that can occur in individual development, or the systematic structure or functional changes in the process." So we are concerned with the potential to change the capacity to modify behavioral function and basically the ability of the nervous system and the organism itself to adapt to the demands of a particular context. Now, the phrase, "particular context," is very important from the point of view of understanding CNS plasticity and function. First of all, what is often seen as a constant that we all take for granted, depending upon our view of reality (i.e., our ideas about how the brain is structured and/or organized), might only be relatively constant from another perspective of neural organization. For example, it is very easy for most of us who are used to the doctrine of cerebral localization to accept the idea of a very specific relationship between the localized site of an injury and its sequalii of behavioral deficits. In neuropsychology, we often take inferences about structure-function relationships as a given fact or firm "truth." Much of neurological research and neurological diagnostics are designed to yield that set of constants (i.e., to support our hypotheses and paradigms we select the appropriate methods and measurements to obtain the "correct" data). But the question becomes then, what happens if structure-function constants are only 'relatively' constant? How then do we localize deficits? What do we treat? What should be our prognosis?

"CONTEXTUAL FACTORS" IN RECOVERY FROM BRAIN DAMAGE:
Serial lesions. Here is one example of how "constant relationships" may change as a function of the context in which these relationships are studied. Since the time of John H. Jackson, neurologists have been aware of the fact that slow-growing injury to the central nervous system does not always result in the same extent of impairment as damage that is inflicted more rapidly. Jackson talked about this in terms of the "momentum of the lesion" effect. In view of examining lesion momentum in a more systematic fashion, we can create slow-growing lesions experimentally to address the question of

constancy and change in the central nervous system. In this context we can ask whether damage inflicted slowly will produce a different behavioral outcome than acute injury - even though the entire brain region is eventually destroyed prior to behavioral evaluation.

To test the momentum of the lesion effect (now better known as the "serial lesion effect"), one must first create a unilateral lesion on one side of the brain, wait a certain amount of time and then remove homologous tissue on the other side, thus creating a bilateral lesion. The subjects with these two-stage lesions are then compared to those with bilateral lesions produced at once and both lesion groups are compared to sham-operated or intact controls. The important point to emphasize is that when testing begins, all of the animals have bilateral brain injury. Now if the lesion is constant, (i.e., extent of damage is the same for both groups of brain-injured subjects), and if the deficits are a constant (as measured by 'standardized' tests), then one would expect that the behavioral outcome of the brain surgery should be the same. But this is not the case. The subjects with several lesions of hippocampus, frontal cortex, and many other CNS regions, perform as well as intact controls, despite the loss of these "key" areas (3,4,5).

The data from one set of studies will serve as an example. We have looked at a number of different kinds of behavioral tests in adult rats with one-stage lesions of the medial frontal cortex. One-stage lesions in this area typically result in long-lasting impairments in spatial abilities. These animals take far longer to learn a spatial alternation task than sham-operated or normal animals. What happens when the same extent of injury is inflicted in several stages? As described in detail elsewhere (3), there are virtually no behavioral deficits. The brain-damaged rats can perform as well as normals, even though the tissue is bilaterally removed. The point that I wish to make is that the issue here is not one of what function(s) is localized in a structure, but what events are occurring before, during or after CNS injury that can facilitate or block functional recovery? What constancies and what variances are occurring in the brain that allow for the kind of sparing we have seen in different experiments using serial lesions to create massive bilateral injuries? This is one example of how long-held views of nervous functions may have to be viewed in a different context; a different 'reality' so-to-speak. One of the primary assumptions we make from the localizationist perspective is that once brain injury is inflicted, the effects are relatively permanent, and that time or how the injury occurs are really not critical factors.

Trophic factors and recovery. In the clinic, it is recognized that various physiological events occurring after injury have a specific time course and may be responsible for the limited 'spontaneous recovery' that one often sees. In fact, in some quarters, it is argued that rehabilitation therapy should not be initiated until all the spontaneous recovery that might occur has been completed. We now know that recovery is not 'spontaneous,' nor is it time itself that mediates the necessary events. Recent evidence suggests that, within hours after injury occurs, the brain begins to produce endogenous, growth promoting substances (trophic factors) that can enhance the survival of neurons that ordinarily die as a result of the injury. These trophic substances are most concentrated at the areas surrounding the injury (6) with a peak period of occurrence at between 7-10 days after the damage has occurred.

In addition to the endogenous production of trophic factors, the injury itself also produces neurotoxic substances which are capable of destroying cells or blocking their regenerative capacities. The trophic substances at the site of the injury work to overcome toxic effects, and we can speculate that the extent of recovery observed following cerebral injury may be the result of 'competition' between trophic and toxic substances working to gain control of neuronal function near the zone of injury. If trophic factors enhance growth and survival over time, then more functional recovery can be expected, whereas if toxic substances predominate, more significant impairments would result. The main point, however, is that both of these competing processes take place over time and that the outcome of brain injury is not a constant. Posttraumatic recovery and/or impairment is rather a complex series of 'environmental' events whose outcome depends on the specific context in which the injury occurs. Site of damage alone is simply not a sufficient predictor of what will happen to the patient at a later time. Also, it is now increasingly likely that these posttraumatic events can be altered by various kinds of therapies, including direct, pharmacological manipulations (e.g., injections of the Nerve Growth Factor directly into the site of the injury--see 7, 8).

In the context of these 'time-dependent processes,' it is interesting to note that there appears to be a 'minimal interval' required for the serial lesion phenomenon to be observed and that this interval corresponds to the period of time required for the maximum release of endogenous trophic substances at the site of the injury (6). Here, we examined how frontal cortex injuries in rats affect spatial learning tasks when the interval between surgical removal is varied from one week to two months.

In this experiment frontal cortex lesions were made with 10, 20, or 30 day intervals between the first and second operations. With 20 and 30 days there is a marked improvement in performance in comparison to animals who are given simultaneous bilateral injury. Even with a 10-day interval there is a smaller deficit in response to brain injury. So, the outcome of injury is not the same even though the final extent of the lesion is the same in all cases. Thus, we have evidence that at both the anatomical/morphological level of analysis and at the behavioral level as well, it is not just the question of damage to the frontal cortex, per se; it is also a question of what are the other variables along with damage itself that lead to sparing of function or severe impairment.

SUBSTITUTION VS. RESTITUTION:

There is yet another issue sometimes overlooked in evaluating recovery from brain damage. Thus, one might ask, when a subject does recover is it substituting new responses for those lost after injury, or is there true "sparing" of the original functions? This is an important question in determining the most appropriate rehabilitation strategies to follow. What is meant by the term 'recovery'? Are rats recovered in the sense that their performance is like that of a normal animal despite the fact that they have no frontal cortex or no motor cortex, or are they simply using a new set of tricks to perform a task that they could not ordinarily or would not ordinarily perform if this part of the brain were intact? Ann Gentile (9) of Columbia University and I examined this question by creating one-or two-stage lesions of the sensorimotor cortex in adult rats who were then required to run back and forth on a narrow, elevated beam in order to obtain water reinforcement. Intact rats quickly learn this task and perform it without any difficulty.

On this task rats with one-stage lesions of motor cortex are initially impaired with respect to rats with lesions made in two stages, despite the fact that all rats eventually learn. What happens if we look more carefully at this phenomenon?

There is a more precise way to measure gait than counting errors on a runway. The animals can be filmed as they cross the narrow platform using a high- speed motion picture camera. Each frame is then used to measure the vertical and horizontal displacement of a hind paw as the animals move along the platform. It is interesting to note is that the momentum of the lesions (i.e., one- or two-stage) determines how the rat's gait is affected. We found that substitution or restitution of function can occur depending upon how the surgery is performed. One-stage rats recovered by substituting a new motor plan for that lost as a result of the injury, while rats with two-stage lesions, of the same extent, had essentially the same movement pattern.

The temporal factors in the recovery process are as important as the damage to the structure because, in both these cases, animals suffered complete bilateral removal of the motor cortex and showed the same extent of neuronal degeneration in the nuclei of the thalamus projecting to the motor cortex. The differences in recovery were not a question of

differential neuronal sparing. The lesions were the
same, yet the behavioral outcomes were quite
different. The findings of the Gentile, et al.
experiments (9) tell us that functional recovery can
be measured in different ways. Thus, on the one
hand, if we are simply interested in whether subjects
can achieve a goal, we could say that all of the rats
'recovered.' If, on the other hand, we are
interested in how subjects recover, a more precise
analysis of the means actually employed to compensate
for the injury would reveal a different outcome. In
the latter case, new responses emerge to compensate
for the movements lost as a result of the injury.
The specific reasons why one- and two-stage injury
lead to different behavioral outcomes still elude
explanation, but, once again, such findings emphasize
the importance of context in describing structure-
function relationships in the central nervous system.

Hormones and recovery. Manipulation of hormonal
state provides yet another example of how "context"
can affect the outcome of brain injury. A number of
years ago, my students and I (4) at Clark University
showed that the serial lesion effect did not seem to
occur in female rats.

What could account for this? At the time we did
not have a good explanation for the fact that removal
of frontal cortex had markedly different effects in
males and females. But this phenomenon did raise the
interesting question of whether there are sex
differences in response to brain injury. Could
ovarian hormones play a role in affecting the outcome
of CNS lesions?

In females, estrogen and progesterone fluctuate as
a function of the estrous cycle and, during the
normal cycle, serum estrogen levels are high and
progesterone is relatively low. If the cycle is

blocked, this relationship is reversed. Despite these hormonal fluctuations, the performance of intact female rats on delayed spatial alternation is normal. Thus, on measures of days to criterion, errors and perseverations, the estrous cycle does not appear to disrupt learned spatial behavior. By providing chronic, mild vaginal stimulation to block the estrous cycling see [10] for details), we can dramatically alter the hormonal status of the female rat. In this 'pseudo-pregnant' state, plasma estrogen levels decrease and progesterone levels increase. Our recent experiments show that reducing levels of estrogen in rats with frontal cortex injury causes a dramatic difference in the outcome of the injury, despite the fact that in normal rats, the estrous cycle has no demonstrable effect on performance. When the same performance is examined after bilateral brain damage, animals with normal estrous cycling are significantly more impaired than when estrous levels are reduced during pseudo-pregnancy.

Once again, data such as these show that the issue of what organismic factors determine the outcome of brain injury is very complex. The point that I want to stress is that whether or not there are species differences in brain function, hormonal (i.e., chemical) factors may play a role in influencing the severity of symptoms and subsequent extent of functional recovery. In a broader sense, individual, organismic and environmental factors must be given more weight in describing the function of a struc-ture or the nature of cognitive and sensory deficits following brain injury.

From the clinical perspective we know that specific symptoms follow damage to specific parts of the nervous system. This lack of plasticity resulting in permanent impairment may be due to the fact that we do not yet know enough about how to initiate or release the plasticity that is inherent in the central nervous system. For example, at the present time there are no available pharmacological treatments for promoting recovery from brain damage. Yet, in the laboratory, we do know that trophic factors such as Nerve Growth Factor and constituents of membranes such as the gangliosides can produce significant functional recovery after brain injury. The administration of trophic substances as a supplement to more traditional therapy can markedly determine the outcome of brain injury and result in varying degrees of sparing or even complete sparing after injury (11, 12).

HOW LONG DOES IT TAKE FOR RECOVERY TO OCCUR?:

Often in a rehabilitation or clinical setting, we tend to use intervals that are very short with respect to the evaluation of brain injury outcome. We believe that there may be a certain degree of spontaneous recovery, and after a relatively short period of time if we do not see any further recovery, the assumption is made that the limits of that plasticity have been attained and there is nothing more that can be done. I think that this is an assumption that really needs to be seriously questioned in light of the examples that have been presented here.

Geschwind (13) recently made the following statement: "There must be many cases in which the capacity for recovery in the central nervous system is latent and revealed only by some other manipulation. <u>Experimenters have only rarely been zealous in their search for the right maneuver</u> (my emphasis)". Most of us working in the area of brain damage in the neurosciences are really not very zealous in our search for the right maneuver to unlock and promote functional recovery. Geschwind also argued that the time needed for recovery in adults may be much longer than in infants, and that we are not really giving enough time and doing enough manipulations over time to promote recovery. He says: "Most neurologists are gloomy about the prognosis of severe adult aphasia after a few weeks and pessimism is reinforced by lack of prolonged follow-up in most cases (my emphasis). I have, however, seen patients severely aphasic for over one year, who then made excellent recovery. One patient returned to work as a salesman, the other as a psychiatrist. Furthermore, there are patients who continue to improve over many years, for example, the patient whose aphasia is still quite evident six years after onset, cleared up substantially by 18 years (p. 3)." Geschwind also pointed out that changes after damage may show great individual variation, which is a factor that never gets much consideration in our search for statistical significance.

In the face of such delayed, but nonetheless extensive, recovery, it makes good sense to ask whether the rate of recovery can be enhanced by rehabilitation (environmental) or pharmacological manipulations (or various combinations of the two approaches). Given that such recovery is possible, the question of treatment then must be based on political and social factors such as cost and commitment of trained specialists. In any case we ought to keep in mind that plasticity and adaptability to brain damage is probabilistic. The outcome, like the outcome of development in general, is not inevitable because all of the environmental and organismic factors that determine and influence recovery from injury are rarely ever systematically manipulated. New approaches to research and therapy are clearly needed in this important domain.

NOT ALL EXAMPLES OF CNS "PLASTICITY" ARE BENEFICIAL:
The extent to which plasticity in the central nervous system occurs will depend upon the coding or bringing together of the appropriate variables at the appropriate time. Here is where we need much more experimental work in both clinical rehabilitation and in basic neuroscience to bring those two fields much closer together.

While I tend to be optimistic about the prospects of promoting CNS recovery, we should remember that there are also negative examples of "plasticity." We cannot be led to believe that every aspect of growth or dynamic change in the central nervous system necessarily needs to be beneficial. For example, while there is neuronal growth in response to injury, not all of it necessarily is adaptive.

Consider neuronal sprouting as an example. Injury-induced sprouting has now been well described but there may be some instances which could lead to maladaptive behavior. The work of Gerald Schneider (14), at the Massachusetts Institute of Technology provides a good example. Schneider has conducted an interesting series of studies in the developing hamster visual system, where the neural pathways from the eye to the lateral geniculate nuclei and superior colliculus are well described. When damage or removal of the superior colliculus is done in the neonatal hamster, some very interesting changes occur. What happens is that optic fibers, which would normally grow into their appropriate collicular targets, do not just die back, they actually reroute into other structures such as deeper layers of the colliculus or even the medial geniculate body.

In addition, if the growing optic fibers do not find the 'appropriate' superior colliculus where it is supposed to be, they grow back, recross the midline and reinnervate the ipsilateral superior colliculus where they compete with the appropriate optic fibers. What happens now? This is a good example of neuronal growth and "plasticity" in response to injury. Fibers do grow--they do not see a superior colliculus for whatever reasons--and they grow back across the midline to compete with normal innervation of the ipsilateral superior colliculus and form new connections there.

Now, if the hamster is presented with a sunflower seed, a normal hamster will take the sunflower seed presented in the appropriate visual field and eat it. But if the hamster is presented with a seed in the damaged visual field with its anomalous crossed and recrossed connections, it will always turn in the opposite direction (away from the seed) because the sunflower seed is apparently perceived in the wrong visual field. This is not adaptive if survival is dependent upon eating sunflower seeds. Here, then, is a good example of neuronal plasticity, but not necessarily a good example of functional recovery. Vision has recovered, but it is not adaptive.

This is an important point for rehabilitation specialists to consider. When one applies "standard operating principles" on an "average", and one does not take the individual variability in context (morphological and environmental) that might be occurring, one might produce organismic responses that are maladaptive.

CONCLUDING REMARKS:

To summarize, there are many, many more examples of plasticity that one can give, but I think we have seen, just from these few examples, that "reality" of central nervous system recovery is very much different than it was just a few years ago. We now know, for example, that fetal brain transplants are being used to promote recovery. We have heard of the possibility that there may be endogenous factors in the central nervous system that can actually promote recovery. Only a few years ago we had no idea of why serial lesions might result in sparing of function. We now know that when neurons are injured, they begin to release endogenous trophic factors. Many of those trophic substances have now been identified and are being employed as experimental therapies for brain injuries.

About 60 years ago, Ramon y Cajal, a Spanish anatomist who won the Nobel Prize, made the statement that: "Once development is ended, the fonts of growth and regeneration dry up irrevocably. In adult centers, the nerve paths are something fixed and mutable. Everything may die; nothing may be regenerated." In the last 10 years, we have come a long way since Ramon y Cajal uttered that dictum, yet, to a considerable extent his dogma and the doctrine of cerebral specificity have thrived. Now we are beginning to recognize that there is indeed far more hope that something can be done to alter the outcome of cerebral injury and to offer its victims a chance for a better quality of life.

REFERENCES

1. Laurence, S., & Stein, D.G. (1978). Recovery after brain damage and the concept of localization of function. In S. Finger (Ed.), Recovery from brain damage: Research and theory (pp. 369-407). New York: Plenum Press.

2. Gollin, E.S. (1981). Development and plasticity. In E.S. Gollin (Ed.), Developmental plasticity: Behavioral and biological aspects of variations in development (p. 231). New York: Academic Press.

3. Stein, D.G., Rosen, J.J., Graziadei, J., Mishkin, D., & Brink, J. (1969). Central nervous system: Recovery of function. Science, 166, 528-530.

4. Stein, D.G. (1974). Some variables influencing recovery of function in the rat. In D.G. Stein, J.J. Rosen, & N. Butters (Eds.), Plasticity and recovery of function in the central nervous system (pp. 373-428). New York: Academic Press.

5. Finger, S., Walbran, B., & Stein D.G. (1973). Brain damage and behavioral recovery: Serial lesion phenomena. Brain Res., 63, 1-18.

6. Cotman, C.W., & Nieto-Sampedro, M. (1985). Progress in facilitating the recovery of function after central nervous system trauma. Ann. N.Y. Acad. Sci., 457, 83-104.

7. Hart, T., Chaimas, N., Moore, R.Y., & Stein, D.G. (1978). Effects of nerve growth factor on behavioral recovery following caudate nucleus lesions in rats. Brain Res. Bull., 3, 245-250.

8. Finger, S., & Stein, D.G. (1982). Drugs and recovery: Nerve growth factor, stimulants and "de-blocking" agents (Chap. 12). In S. Finger, & D.G. Stein, Brain damage and recovery: Research and clinical perspectives (pp. 227-256). New York: Academic Press.

9. Gentile, A.M., Green, S., Nieburgs, A., Schmeltzer, W., & Stein, D.G. (1978). Disruption and recovery of locomotor and manipulating behavior following cortical lesions in rats. Behav. Biol., 22, 417-455.

10. Attella, M., Nattinville, A., & Stein, D.G. (in press). Hormonal state affects recovery from frontal cortex lesions in adult female rats. Behav. & Neural. Biol.

11. Stein, D.G. (1980). Functional recovery from brain damage following treatment with nerve growth factor. In M.W. van Hof, & G. Mohn (Eds.), Functional recovery from brain damage (pp. 423-444). Amsterdam: Elsevier, N. Holland.

12. Stein, D.G., & Sabel, B. (Eds.). (in press).
    Pharmacological approaches to the treatment of
    brain and spinal cord injury. New York: Plenum
    Press.
13. Geschwind, N. (1985). Mechanisms of change
    after brain lesions. Ann. N.Y. Acad. Sci., 457,
    1-13.
14. Schneider, G.E., & Jhaveri, S.R. (1974).
    Neuroanatomical correlates of spared or altered
    function after brain lesions in the newborn
    hamster. In D.G. Stein, J.J. Rosen, & N.
    Butters (Eds.), Plasticity and recovery of
    function in the central nervous system
    (pp. 65-110). New York: Academic Press.

2

NEUROPHARMACOLOGY AND BRAIN DAMAGE
D. Nathan Cope
The National Rehabilitation Hospital
Washington, D.C. 20010 - 2949
U. S. A.

Until recently there has been little in the
scientific literature regarding the psychopharmacologic
treatment of traumatic brain injury (TBI). To some
extent this is due to the late clinical recognition of
TBI as an important and distinct syndrome from a
neurobehavioral (as well as a neurosurgical) perspective. A preliminary nosology of TBI has not been ade-
quately developed to allow necessary syndrome dis-
crimination in studies of drug effect. For TBI studies,
there has, to date, been a lack of double-blind techniques.

The brain is a specifically organized organ
comprised of highly precise distributions of discrete
neurotransmitter systems. Brain injury is not a single
entity, but rather a collection of distinct syndromes
(which occur with greater or lesser frequency in any
population of traumatic closed head injury patients),
each of which has its own presumably distinct disturbance of neurotransmitter function. Minor head injury
may consist primarily of shearing lesions of long
axonal tracts (1,2), which includes a proportion of the
ascending catecholaminergic projections from the lower
brainstem area. It has been reported that there are
routine deficiencies of catecholaminergic and seroto-
nergic metabolites in cerebrospinal fluid of TBI
patients, which vary depending upon the various ana-

tomical characteristics of the original brain injury
(3,4). Even purely focal CNS injuries are known to have
neurotransmitter effects far beyond the site of the
injury. The condition of TBI has a varying profile of
affected neurotransmitter systems from case to case.

We are far from being able to specify the clinical
effects in any individual case. This complex mixture of
determinants makes it very difficult to be confident
about any prediction of efficacy for a particular drug
in any behavioral or psychological syndrome with any
individual TBI patient.

It is encouraging to note, however, an emerging
interest and appreciation within the psychopharmacologic field for the unique therapeutic challenges of
TBI. This is reflected in an increasing number of
reports of psychopharmacologic interventions for the
behavioral problems of TBI of increasingly sophisti-
cated design (5,6).

TBI patients have a wide spectrum of neurological,
perceptual, motor, language, cognitive, behavioral, and
affective deficits. Specific neuropsychologic treatment
approaches (7) as well as elaborate systems of rehabilitation care (8) have been developed to manage the
various syndromes.

THEORETICAL ISSUES

At a more theoretical level there are further
issues to be considered in the decision to use psychopharmacological agents to treat the TBI patient. These
drugs act primarily by modifying the underlying neurotransmitter physiology of the brain. It appears, however, that the brain may have characteristic responses
to alterations which is basically a homeostatic process. To an extent not yet clearly defined there is a
tendency for the CNS to alter its own neurophysiologic
activity to counter any exogenous effects of neuroactive drugs. The risk exists that these responses

from the brain will have non-therapeutic consequences. The most common and the most prominent clinical example of this is tardive dyskinesia.

Tardive dyskinesia is a syndrome of gradual development of involuntary movement, and is associated with the use of the antipsychotic medications. The incidence of this condition can be distressingly high (9), and while most clearly related to the total lifetime dose of the drug, can occur within a very short interval after drug initiation. Tardive dyskinesia in many cases may be irreversible. A 1985 American Psychiatric Association statement on tardive dyskinesia concludes that the use of neuroleptics for organic brain syndromes is indicated only for short-term management (6 months) (10).

Unfortunately, many agitated TBI patients end up on antipsychotics not only acutely, but for many years, particularly when they reside in institutional settings or are not in active treatment programs. It is becoming a malpractice situation if one treats patients with antipsychotics in a negligent (i.e. non-indicated) manner or fails to examine for this type of movement disorder at periodic intervals. What should be clearly appreciated by clinicians is that evidence exists which supports only a limited role for the use of neuroleptics in organic brain conditions. This is not simply a theoretical medical-legal danger; it has been suggested that the next major malpractice crisis in the U.S. will be concerned with just such non-indicated use of these drugs, with the consequent emergence of tardive dyskinesia (11).

An aspect of the use of these neuroactive drugs that is not generally considered is their possible influence on the actual recovery from the brain lesion itself. There is evidence that certain neuroactive drugs may either enhance or retard recovery from

neurological lesions. A series of animal studies by
Feeney and associates (12,13) investigated recovery
from a sensory-motor cortical ablation in rats and
cats. The rate of recovery from hemiplegia following
ablation is measured by means of a balance beam task.
Amphetamine given in a single physiologic dose shortly
after induction of the cortical lesion produces a consistent and statistically significant acceleration of
recovery. Conversely, a single dose of haloperidol,(a
catecholaminergic blocking agent) rather than amphetamines (a catecholamine agonist) induces a prolonged delay before recovery of motor function occurs
(12). These findings have been replicated with contusion, as well as, ablation models of brain injury
(13). Even beyond the acute post-injury phase the use
of catecholaminergic blocking agents may increase
expressed neurologic dysfunction. Van Hassalt demonstrated that after recovery from experimentally induced
sensory-motor deficit in animals the administration of
a single dose of haloperidol would reinstitute hemiplegia. These responses occurred repetitively each time
the drug was administered (14). In terms of human
studies related to this animal work a recent report
indicated that in a group of aphasic patients, use of
haloperidol in the clinical management was associated
with a poorer than predicted recovery from their
aphasic disorder (15). This naturalistic study had no
controls, but nevertheless offers some indication that
the theoretical risks suggested by the above animal
work may have clinical significance.

In summary, there is evidence available that
suggests that the use of agents which affect neurotransmitter activity in CNS will have not only immediate behavioral effects, but also the potential for
influencing level or rate of recovery from CNS injury.
Clinicians may be inducing an unperceived additional

neuropathological burden on patients with brain injury, by reflexively relying upon neuropharmacologic treat- ments for the management of what may be transient behavioral disorders. Obviously, more study is required in this area.

CLINICAL CONSIDERATIONS

As a result of the clinical complexity of TBI and lack of data there are significant problems with determining in clinical settings what might be ap- propriate neuropharmacologic approaches to brain injury. It is an unfortunately common circumstance that psychiatric consultations to TBI rehabilitation pro- grams are not perceived as generally helpful in manag- ing these patients. Such consultation is usually requested for a typical TBI patient who, having been in coma, is now recovering consciousness and is severe- ly agitated, assaulting the nursing or therapy staff, sleeping only a few minutes at a time, and who may be destructive to hospital equipment. The psychiatric question is usually how to best manage these severe behavioral disturbances.

It may not be totally unfair to characterize the current psychiatric approach to this disruptive patient with organic brain syndrome as follows: determine whether the patient is suffering from a treatable organic condition such as vitamin deficiency, metal intoxication, occult mass lesion, or infection, etc. If not, minimize overstimulation and maximize orienting cues, (e.g. leave a light on at night, etc.). Finally these approaches proving ineffective, prescribe a high potency antipsychotic neuroleptic.

It is appropriate, given the current level of uncertainty, to first do no harm through unnecessary or ill considered drug interventions. A search for pre- cipitating stimuli such as infection, pain, overly stimulating environments, and overly demanding requests

from the treatment team, should be looked for and
eliminated before resorting to pharmacologic approaches. When pharmacologic treatment is begun use of
single case methodology is appropriate. However in
practice, if careful attention is not given to application, single case methods are seldom actually employed.

One gets multiple measures of the target (and
important adaptive) behaviors and evaluates whether
changes in these behaviors coincide with institution of
drug treatment. It is essential that in addition to
looking at target symptoms, an assessment be done to
determine if drug treatment suppresses adaptive behaviors. For this, there must be a broad range of measures taken, not simply a frequency count of assaults.
Ideally, measures of mobility and self-care capacities,
as well as, various psychometric measures, such as
arousal, information processing, and memory need
assessment. In many cases there is a trade-off of lost
adaptive capacity for gained behavioral control, and
evaluation of this trade-off requires a baseline, a
treatment, and a placebo, or washout, phase. The most
common error is to simply institute a treatment phase,
and measure only the target behavior. Speaking practi-
cally, however, there are some problems (at least in
the U.S.) in following this ideal format precisely.
Utilization review constraints tend to prevent maintenance of patients in a treatment program long enough
to use all of the aspects of this approach. At the very
least drug treatment and withdrawal phase are needed to
demonstrate that drug treatment is actually the responsible agent for whatever improvement is observed.

Psychopharmacologic approaches might be considered for four general clinical problems after TBI. The
first is the pharmacologic approach to the comatose or
poorly aroused patient. A variety of drugs that in

general are agonists of the catecholaminergic system,
are felt to perhaps improve the responsiveness of
patients with severely depressed arousal levels secondary to TBI and other CNS pathology (16,17). Such
agents as amphetamines, methylphenidate, and L-Dopa are
suggested by anecdotal studies to improve the arousal
level of patients in either a comatose or a stuporous
state. Some clinicians are routinely using these drugs
in the rehabilitation setting to promote increased
arousal (18). Although of great interest and potential
usefulness, a great deal of further evaluation is
required before this pharmacologic approach can be a
routine component of clinical care.

A second area is for presumed affective disorder,
i.e. depression. In brain injured patients it has
generally been difficult clinically to ascertain
whether certain signs and symptoms, such as the lack of
verbal behaviors, or vegetative disturbances such as
sleep, appetite, and sexual disruption are reflective
of a primary depressive disorder or of more straightforward neurologic deficits. There is evidence appearing from stroke patients with similar "depressive"
phenomena, that a form of depression does in fact occur
in brain injured patients (19). These patients respond
to tricyclics roughly, as well as, non-neurologically
impaired depressives (20). It is conceivable that TBI
patients who "look depressed" may also have a similar
gratifying response to standard antidepressants.

The third area in which medications are considered
as possible interventions is in remediating the basic
cognitive deficits which follow brain injury. At the
risk of oversimplification, these deficits are felt to
lie principally in at least three areas; memory, attention and information processing. Cognitive enhancement
or remediation of these deficits by pharmacologic
agents has a small literature, and one that again

derives more from a variety of associated organic brain syndromes than from TBI itself.

Most widely studied are the cognitive declines associated with senile, Alzheimer's or alcoholic induced dementias (21,22). Cholinergic agonists, anticholinesterase agents, and certain neuropeptides have been used in attempts to improve memory function. Attention and information processing have been treated by catecholamine agonists, such as amphetamines or methylphenidate, and by a variety of other neurotransmitter interventions. A comprehensive review is available (23).

Recent reports of attempts to remediate these cognitive dysfunctions in TBI suggest in some cases a rather successful result (24). This area of psychopharmacologic intervention is also still in the very early phases of investigation, and while these are promising approaches there are no definitely effective pharmacologic mechanisms to improve cognition after TBI. At the same time it is clear that any effective approach, when developed, will have tremendous beneficial impact upon a large group of TBI victims. It is difficult to conceptualize a more significant area of need for valid study.

The fourth and last common problem which often elicits psychopharmacologic intervention is quite different. This is the management of the agitated or assaultive patient. This problem is certainly by far the most frequent situation which elicits psychopharmacologic management in clinical practice. It is a sometimes poorly appreciated clinical fact that "as head injured patients get better, they get worse". Early after injury, the comatose patient usually is not an unmanageable problem in terms of his or her behavior. As the patient regains full arousal, cognition and judgement characteristically lag behind motor recovery, so that the patient is frequently confused, irritable, frightened, emotionally labile, and impervious to normal explanation, reassurance, or counseling. These patients can be extremely difficult to manage, and not infrequently become impossible to control within usual clinical programs. If they are kept on the usual rehabilitation unit they are ultimately almost always sedated, often to the point of stupor, with obvious detrimental effects upon their rehabilitation program.

Patients alternatively may be transferred to locked psychiatric facilities. The psychodynamic, "therapeutic milieu", or other traditionally oriented approaches of such units prove ineffective for these "demented" patients. Since most locked psychiatric units do not have rehabilitation nursing or therapy capabilities, patients in such settings are denied needed treatment. The problem tends to be not only a very difficult, but a very common one at certain stages of recovery from TBI. The behavioral problems of this phase are a stimulus to the clinical team to solicit psychopharmacologic management.

Given that this is a very common problem and the uncertainty about the sum of the effects of the use of these medications how is this patient treated? What does a positive response to medication mean in these cases? The number of assaults or level of agitation may be decreased, but important additional questions include what adaptive behaviors are affected?

It should, for completeness, be pointed out too that there are significant non-medical influences upon the decision to use medications in clinical settings which should be appreciated. It is known that in nursing home and institutional settings the majority of patients with significant organic impairment tend to be chronically maintained on psychotropic medications (25,

26). There are pressures upon the treating physicians
and institutional administrations favoring the use of
medications. An economic incentive exists to control
behavior by non-labor intensive means. Controlled
behavior programs can manage the majority of behavior-
ally disturbed patients without recourse to medications; that this does not occur is probably not because
of any deficiency of technical information on the part
of clinicians or administrators, but rather due to the
expense of such intervention. It is less expensive to
write a prescription than to organize a complete team
for behavioral management. Governments have an interest
also (at least the U.S.) in promoting, or at least not
discouraging, pharmacologic management. A fixed reimbursement rate is usually provided for the management
of most long-term care patients. Any treatment that
increases the cost of care for these patients is going
to be resisted at some administrative or reimbursement
level.

Taking this scientific uncertainty and competing
economic pressure into consideration, there still
occurs the necessity to make some selection of agents
when drug intervention is necessary. A review of the
rationale and supporting evidence for use of the most
indicated classes of drugs for intervention in the
behavioral disturbances of TBI follows.

Neuroleptics

The most frequently advocated class of drug for
management of the agitated or aggressive organic brain
damaged or demented patient is the neuroleptic. These
drugs are essentially universally recommended by
psychiatric and neurologic texts. In spite of a massive
amount of controlled investigation of the efficacy of
these drugs on traditional psychiatric diagnoses such
as schizophrenia, very little controlled evidence is
available regarding the effectiveness in the organic

conditions. Helms reviewed the literature on the
effectiveness of these drugs for dementia and determined 21 adequate studies that provided only modest
support for their efficacy (27). Similar lack of strong
evidence of neuroleptic effectiveness for dementia
patients has been reported by Barnes who found only a
modest efficacy, but also a strong placebo effect
(28).

These uncertain results of effectiveness are also
available for the behavioral disturbances of the
mentally retarded (29). General restraint is urged in
the use of neuroleptics in these circumstances due to
the increasingly recognized toxicity associated with
their use (30). It is instructive to appreciate that
there are essentially no controlled studies of the
effect of antipsychotics in TBI. Antipsychotics may not
be the drugs of first choice for TBI. In most cases
they produce a general suppression of behavior and are
particularly undesirable in TBI due to their secondary
effects. Also they interfere with processes we are
trying to facilitate in a TBI rehabilitation setting.

For example, these antipsychotics are by and
large epileptogenic, and their use would predispose
the development of seizures in any population of
treated patients (31). Again this is a particularly undesirable feature in TBI with its high predisposition
to epilepsy. The characteristic is also true of most
of the anti-depressants.

Another associated effect of the antipsychotics
and the tricyclics is a strong anticholinergic action.
Interference with the cholinergic system prevents
encoding of immediate into long-term memory (32,33).
The typical TBI patient has as one principal functional
deficit this very inability to encode ongoing events
into long-term memory. He or she often cannot learn
such simple facts as the names of the treating team

members, or learn the name of the facility in which he is receiving care. If this patient is put on medication with significant anticholinergic effects, this has a potential to impair memory further and make the rehabilitation and learning process more difficult. TBI patients who have been treated with haloperidol during their rehabilitation have significantly increased duration of post-traumatic amnesia than matched patients who did not receive such medication (34).

In conclusion, there are situations where antipsychotics may be specifically indicated for TBI. They appear to be particularly effective if the clinical picture involves symptomatology similar to the classic primary signs of schizophrenia, such as hallucinations, paranoid ideations, and ideas of reference. In these situations the antipsychotics may have a particularly specific effect and are probably indicated. The contraindications to their use increase with the length of time. Certainly long-term use to suppress chronic behavioral disturbance without efforts to define other effective approaches (either behavioral or pharmacologic) is not appropriate.

Antidepressants

As discussed above, the question of depression in organic brain lesions has been difficult for psychiatry because of the confounding problems of neurologic deficits obscuring some of the very fundamental biologic signs of depression. Only recently have adequate studies been reported that indicate what "appears" to be depression in the brain injured patient is a response to tricyclics similar to primary depressive disorders (19,20).

A second rationale relating to the use of antidepressants in TBI is the concept of the attention deficit disorders (ADD). This syndrome originally comprised children who have problems with distractibility and sustained attention. They tend to be impulsive, show aggression and sociopathy. The syndrome now, however, is known to persist into adulthood. The clinical symptoms of this condition are reliably ameliorated by antidepressants, which are usually recommended as a back-up approach after the stimulants, methylphenidate and the amphetamines, have proven ineffective. In many series of hyperkinetic children there is a large subset of members with definite histories of TBI. Often the symptomatology of the hyperkinesis will derive precisely from the date of the brain injury itself. The behavioral and cognitive symptomatology of brain injury is very similar to the symptomatology seen in ADD. Particularly with mild or moderate brain injured patients, the similarity of the distractibility, impulsivity, and irritability is very striking. The hypothesis is that both antidepressants and stimulant medications may be as useful for these problems in TBI, as they are for ADD. Several recent studies in TBI lend support to this concept. Effective management of impulsive, agitated TBI patients have been reported by Mysiw and Jackson who have treated these patients with amitriptyline (35,36).

Minor Tranquilizers

The minor tranquilizers are often recommended for the psychopharmacologic management of agitation in emergency situations where there is lack of diagnostic clarity on the etiology of the disturbance. This approach is based in part on the very high safety margin of the benzodiazepines. They do not have the epileptogenic or anticholinergic potential of the antipsychotics or the cardiotoxic qualities of the antidepressants. The benzodiazepines have a general reputation as effective "antiaggressive" agents. Any such effect has been shown to be species and situation specific (37).

Benzodiazepines may, in fact, exacerbate agitation (38). They may be the most appropriate choice for the acute behavioral emergency to establish control quickly and safely. It should be understood that this use is a temporary emergency management intervention. The benzodiazepines do not appear to have a clear indication for the long-term management of behavioral difficulties following TBI. These drugs are cortical suppressants, and therefore impair the arousal and cognitive processes in an often unacceptable manner (39).

Another situation one encounters regarding benzodiazepines is the common case where they are utilized as antispasticity agents. The risk/benefit aspect of the antispasticity treatment has to be considered in relation to the trade-off between the benefit of reducing spasticity and the associated cognitive impairment accompanying it.

Lithium

Lithium is a usually rarely considered possibility for the management of the agitated TBI patient. Traditionally this drug has been indicated for the treatment of primary bipolar disease. However, it is quite well demonstrated that with certain specific CNS lesions a true, but secondary, manic psychosis appears. The available reports of secondary mania concern a variety of types of organic brain syndromes, including neoplasm, CVA's, trauma, etc. (40). This secondary manic psychosis appears to be also responsive to lithium (41). Many of these series of patients more generally classified as organic brain syndrome include patients whose secondary mania derives from TBI (42,43). Results from lithium use in the aggressive or agitated head injury patient appears to be effective (44).

In addition, there appears to be an attribute of lithium which has a mood stabilizing or antiaggressive

effect even in the absence of any actual manic syndrome. A number of studies in various diagnostic
groups, including mentally retarded children and
aggressive or violent incarcerated prisoners have
demonstrated that the use of lithium, independent of
any manic depressive diagnosis, will reduce aggressive
and irritable episodes (45,46). Many individuals
within these populations also appear to have suffered
TBI.

Anticonvulsants

The importance of the anticonvulsants in clinical
practice is their frequent use in TBI for seizure
management or prophylaxis. A great number of traumatic
brain injury patients are treated with anticonvulsants,
usually phenytoin, phenobarbital or carbamazepine.

Phenytoin and phenobarbital have now been clearly
shown to significantly impair cognition and behavior
independent of any influence of seizure frequency
(47,48). Statistical drop in various intellectual
measures such as Wechsler IQ scores among patients
occur with these drugs. If one removes the drug, a
reliable and reproducible increase in cognitive function results. The drug induced impairment occurs in a
dose related manner that is significant even at therapeutic blood levels.

The first issue, in regard to anticonvulsants, is
that there is a cognitive price associated with the use
of this class of medication, at least with phenobarbital and phenytoin. Any opportunity to manage TBI patients by avoiding these drugs is probably worthwhile.
It has not been demonstrated that the use of anticonvulsants for the prophylaxis of epilepsy is useful, and
therefore this indication should no longer be considered valid.

Carbamazepine appears to have substantially
different qualities than phenytoin or phenobarbital in

terms of its non-anticonvulsant effects. It has been
suggested that carbamazepine does not produce cognitive
impairment at therapeutic levels. Some studies have
indicated that the use may in fact improve mood,
attention, or information processing (49). Carbamazepine appears to be the anticonvulsive of choice in
brain injury since it produces less cognitive impairment than the other varieties of anticonvulsants. A
second perspective on anticonvulsants, and carbamazepine in particular, has to do with the syndrome termed
temporal lobe epilepsy or limbic system epilepsy
(50,51). This syndrome is characterized by seizure
occurrences of automatic motor and behavioral manifes-
tations which sometimes include assaultiveness, at-
tacks, and violence, and is known to have a relationship to brain injury. This concept is a complex and
controversial area in neurology and psychiatry, and
while the existence of such events appears certain, it
is unclear how frequently they occur. They are probably
rare phenomena and not usually involved in the behavioral problems of most TBI patients.

Associated with temporal lobe epilepsy is the
concept of temporal or limbic lobe instability. A
postulated interictal personality develops. Patients
with prolonged seizure disorders have been noted to
progressively develop distinctive personality disturbances. This personality is characterized by trucu-
lence, irritability, and tendency toward assaultiveness. The reported use of anticonvulsants in these
cases, independent of any overt clinically manifested
seizure disorder per se, will nevertheless produce
clinical improvement in these problematic areas of
behavior. Carbamazepine has been suggested as particularly effective in reducing the symptomatology of this
putative interictal personality process (52,53). A

similar use for carbamazepine has been postulated for
the analogous behavior following TBI.

Stimulants

The rationale for the use of stimulants (amphetamines and methylphenidate) in traumatic head injury
is very similar to that discussed previously for the
antidepressants and ADD. These agents may reduce
agitation which is secondary to cognitive deficits,
and improve arousal, vigilance, attention and secondary agitation. There is an increasing literature on
the efficacy of this class of drugs on the disturbances
following brain injury (54,55,56,57).

Beta-blockers

The beta-blockers are the final class of drugs to
be mentioned. Propranolol is the most prominent and
frequently used member of this class. These drugs
inhibit the beta-adrenergic system both centrally and
peripherally. A variety of clinical studies have been
reported in the last five or six years which have
demonstrated the response of certain numbers of agitated and assaultive brain impaired patients, including
patients with TBI, both acute and chronic, to beta
blockers (58,59,60,61). This response has occurred
after the failure of multiple other agents such as the
antipsychotics, antidepressants, and lithium. Dosages
which are effective appear to at times be quite high
(over 1000 mg/day of propranolol). The beta-blockers
appear to be a feasible alternative to other more
usually considered drugs.

CONCLUSION

There are a number of possible effective psychopharmacologic treatments possible for TBI. Usually
accepted choices may not be most appropriate. It is
regretable that so little has been done to evaluate
the benefits and dangers of psychopharmacologic treatment of TBI. At the same time, it is exciting that

investigations in the future may produce a tremendous improvement in our ability to help the sufferers of this condition. The fact that the psychopharmacologic treatment of head injury is a "terra incognita" is both its tragedy and its promise.

REFERENCES

1.   Stritch, S.J. Lancet 2: 443-448, 1961.
2.   Levin, H.S., Handel, S.F., Goldman, A.M. et al. Arch.Neurol. 42: 963-968, 1985.
3.   Van Woerkom, T.C. Lancet 1: 812-813, 1977.
4.   Robinson, R.G., Bloom, F.E. Biol. Psychiatry 12: 669-680, 1977.
5.   Cope, D.N. J. Head Trauma Rehabil. 2(4), 1987.
6.   Cope, D.N., In: Closed Head Injury: Medical Rehabilitation (Ed.S.Berrol), In Preparation.
7.   Grimm, B.H. and Bleiberg, J. In: Handbook of Clinical Neuropsychology, Vol. II. New York: John Wiley and Sons, 1986, pp. 495- 560.
8.   Cope, D.N. Sem.Neurol. 5: 212-220, 1985.
9.   Simpson, GM. Pi, E.H. and Sramek, J. J. Hosp.Comm. Psychia. 37: 362-370, 1986.
10. APA Statement on Tardive Dyskinesia (no author) Hosp.Comm.Psychia. 36: 902, 1985.
11. Appelbaum, P.S., Schaffner, K. and Meisel, A. Am.J. Psychia. 142: 806-810, 1985.
12. Feeney, D.M., Gonzalez, A., Law, W.A., et al. Science 217: 855-857, 1982.
13. Feeney, D.M., Bailey, B.Y., Boyeson, M.G. et al. Brain Injury 1: 27-32, 1987.
14. Van Hassalt, P., Neuropharm. 12: 245-247, 1973.
15. Porch, B., Wyckes, J., et al. Soc. Neurosci. (Abstract) May 1, 1985.
16. Higashi, K., Sakata, Y., Hatano, S., et al. J. Neurol.Neurosurg.Psychiat. 40: 876-885, 1977.
17. Chandra, B. Eur.Neurol. 17: 265-270, 1978.
18. Mayer, N.P. Personal Communication. Moss Rehabilitation Hospital, Philadelphia, 1987.
19. Robinson, R.G., Starr, L.B., Lipsey, J.R. et al.J. Nerv.Ment.Dis. 173: 221-226, 1985.
20. Lipsey, J.R., Robinson, R.G. and Pearlson, G.D. Lancet 1: 297-300, 1984.
21. Gottfries, G.C., Clinical.Neuropharm. 10: 313-329, 1987.
22. Reisberg, B., Ferris, S.H. and Gerson, S. Am.J. Psychia. 138: 593-598, 1981.
23. Wolkowitz, O.M., Tinklenberg, J.R. and Weingartner, H. Neuropsychobiol. 14: 133-156, 1985.

24. Evans, R.W., Gualtieri, T.C. and Patterson, D. J., Nerv.Ment.Dis. 1987, In Press.
25. Rango, J. NEJM 307: 883-890, 1982.
26. Waxman, H.M., Klein, M. and Carner, E.A. Hosp. Comm.Psychia. 36: 886-887, 1985.
27. Helms, P.M. J.Am.Geriatr.Soc. 33: 206-209, 1985.
28. Barnes, R.: Am.J.Psychia. 139: 1170-1174, 1982.
29. Rothmann, CB., Chusid, E. and Giannini, M.J. N.Y. Stat.J.Med. 79: 709-715, 1979.
30. Settle, E.C. J. Clin.Psychia. 44: 440-448, 1983.
31. Logothetis, J. Neurol. 17: 869-877, 1967.
32. Sadeh, M., Braham, J. and Modan, M. Arch.Neurol. 39: 666-669, 1982.
33. Tune, L.E., Strauss, M.E. and Lew, M.F. Am.J.Psychia. 139: 1460-1462, 1982.
34. Rao, N., Jellinek, H.M. and Woolston, D.C. Arch. Phys. Med.Rehabil. 66: 30-34, 1985.
35. Mysiw, W.J. and Jackson, R.D. J.Head Trauma Rehabil. 2: In Press, 1987.
36. Jackson, R.D., Corrigan, J.D. and Arnett, J.A. Arch. Phys.Med.Rehabil. 66: 180-181, 1985.
37. Rodgers, R.J. and Waters, A.J. Neurosci.Biobehav. Rev. 9: 21-35, 1985.
38. Strahan, A., Rosenthal, J., Kaswan, M., et al. Am.J.Psychia. 142: 859-861, 1985.
39. Cole, J.O., Haskell, D.S. and Orzack, H. McLean Hosp. J. 6: 46-74, 1981.
40. Jampala, V.C. and Abrams, R. Am.J.Psychia. 140: 1197-1199, 1983.
41. Williams, K.H. and Goldstein, G. Am.J.Psychia. 138: 800-803, 1979.
42. Shukla, S., Cook, B.L., Mukherjee, S., et al. Am.J.Psychia. 144: 93-96, 1987.
43. Reiss, H., Schwirtz, C.E. and Klermann, G.L. Am.J. Psychia. 48: 29-30, 1987.
44. Glenn, M.B. and Joseph, A.B. J.Head Trauma Rehabil. 2: In Press, 1987.
45. De Paulo, J.R., Correa, E.I. and Folstein, M.F. Biol. Psychia. 18: 1093-1097, 1983.
46. Sheard, M.H., Marini, J.L., Bridges, C.I., et al. Am.J.Psychia. 133: 1409-1413, 1976.
47. Trimble, M.R. Epilepsia 24: (suppl) 555-563, 1983.
48. Fischbacher, E. Brit.Med.J. 285: 423-424, 1982.
49. Evans, R.W. and Gualtieri, C.T. Clin. Neuropharmacol. 8: 221-241, 1985.
50. Pincus, J.H. Neurol. 30: 304-305, 1980.
51. Devinsky, O. and Bear, D. Am.J.Psychiatry 141: 651- 656, 1984.
52. Garbutt, J.C. and Loosen, P.T. Am.J.Psychia. 140: 1363-1364, 1983.
53. Mattes, J.A. Lancet 2: 1164-1165, 1984.
54. Evans, R.W., Gualtieri, T.C. and Patterson, D.R. J. Nerv.Ment.Dis. 175: 106-110, 1987.

55. Lipper, S. and Tuchman, M.M. J.Nerv.Ment.Dis. <u>162</u>: 366-371, 1976.
56. Frances, A. and Jensen, P.S. Hosp.Comm.Psychia. <u>36</u>: 711-713, 1985.
57. Evans, R.W. and Gualtieri, C.T. J.Head Trauma Rehabil. <u>2</u>: In Press, 1987.
58. Yudofsky, S.C. Am.J.Psychia. <u>141</u>: 114-115, 1984.
59. Elliott, F.A. Ann.Neurol. <u>1</u>: 489-491, 1977.
60. Ratey, J.J. Am.J.Psychia. <u>140</u>: 1356-1357, 1983.
61. Mattes, J.A. Am.J.Psychia. <u>142</u>: 1108-1109, 1985.

3

CURRENT RESEARCH IN THE NEUROPSYCHOLOGICAL REHABILITATION
OF BRAIN DAMAGE

LANCE E. TREXLER,

Center for Neuropsychological Rehabilitation and CNR
Research Institute, 8925 North Meridian Street,
Indianapolis, IN 46260, USA

A proliferation of rehabilitation services has
attempted to meet some of the clinical needs of the brain
injured population. Significant progress has been made,
clinically and scientifically, over the last decade.
Nonetheless, an integration of scientific findings with
clinical practice would appear to be particularly
important at the developmental stage in which
neuropsychological rehabilitation currently resides.
Trexler (1) has reviewed a number of professional issues
which bear significantly on the practice of
neuropsychological rehabilitation, some of which include a
re-examination of our assumptions about the nature of
neuropsychological function and methods of clinical
practice and research.

The focus of the present work is to review some of
the research in the neuropsychological rehabilitation,
with specific reference to how certain assumptions
influence research methods. Further, the present work
will review some of the research conducted at the Center
for Neuropsychological Rehabilitation, which emphasizes an
examination of the determinants of recovery approach to
studying neuropsychological rehabilitation. Finally, the
present work will discuss some of the important clinical
issues in the rehabilitation of brain damage which have
yet to be addressed in systematic research.

RESEARCH IN THE REHABILITATION OF NEUROPSYCHOLOGICAL DEFECTS FOLLOWING BRAIN DAMAGE

Recent research has predominantly focused on the rehabilitation of attention, memory and visuospatial defects following brain damage. The clinical practice of evaluating and treating these functions, as well as our research methodologies, has followed from diverging philosophical assumptions about the nature of neuropsychological function and its recovery.

Trexler (2) has described reductionistic and dynamic approaches to neuropsychological rehabilitation, which follow from corresponding assumptions about methods of evaluating neuropsychological function. It is not surprising that rehabilitative methodology has followed from our testing and examination methods, in that the history of clinical neuropsychology was founded on evaluation. Trexler (2) has described diverging approaches to neuropsychological examination as ranging from psychometric and statistical to theoretical and clinical approaches. Table 1 reviews the characteristics of these two approaches.

TABLE 1

DIVERGING ASSUMPTIONS IN THE DEFINITION
OF NEUROPSYCHOLOGICAL FUNCTION

PSYCHOMETRIC-STATISTICAL	THEORETICAL-CLINICAL
-diagnostic reliability	-descriptive
and validity	-hypothesis testing
-normative reference	-qualification of defect
-standardized administration	-dynamic and continuous
-quantitative analysis	changes in
-"test-defined" deficits	functioning
-linear gradient of impairment	-multi-dimensional and
	interactive

Neuropsychological examination based upon
psychometric and statistical assumptions emphasize
quantification of function as a means to determine level
of functioning, typically on a uni-dimensional gradient
ranging from above average to impaired, as compared with a
normative reference group. Many of these
neuropsychological procedures were developed so as to
reliably discriminate brain damaged from non-brain damaged
groups. Theoretical and clinical approaches to
neuropsychological examination have contrastingly
emphasized qualifying the underlying neuropsychological
defects, particularly in terms of the individual factors
which influence the patient's functioning on a given
neuropsychological test. Consequently, the continuous
interaction of neuropsychological functions is emphasized.
The examination methodology therefore proceeds in a
relatively unique manner for each patient, testing serial
hypotheses about the quality of the patient's
neuropsychological defects. These two approaches can best

be dichotomized by the work of Reitan and Davison (3) in the United States with that of Luria (4) and Christensen (5) in the Soviet Union and Denmark, respectively.

As stated, these diverging approaches have carried forward to methods of neuropsychological rehabilitation, and hence research methodology. Corresponding to methods of neuropsychological evaluation, Trexler (2) has described reductionistic and dynamic methods of neuropsychological rehabilitation. Reductionistic methods emphasize a fractionization of components of neuropsychological function, usually viewing components as hierarchially organized. This approach assumes that through restoration of a hierarchially related series of components there is an additivity, such that the 'parts equal the whole.' Rehabilitation methods are standardized given the presence of psychometrically defined neuropsychological defects. The goal of the rehabilitation methods is to enhance functioning to some normative level. The dynamic approach has some history in aphasia rehabilitation, as described by Basso, Capitani and Vignolo (6). Dynamic approaches to rehabilitation emphasize continuously modifying the intervention according to multi-dimensional influences on the patient's functioning. These influences originate in the patient's environment, occur as a function of physiological mechanisms of recovery and the patient's psychological and emotional functioning, to name a few. Therefore, a dynamic approach to neuropsychological rehabilitation emphasizes flexibility in the treatment regime (in vitro), in consideration of the functional adaptation of the patients in their natural environment (in vivo). Table 2 summarizes the characteristics of these two schools of neuropsychological rehabilitation.

TABLE 2

DIVERGING APPROACHES TO NEUROPSYCHOLOGICAL REHABILITATION

REDUCTIONISTIC	DYNAMIC
-components of function and fractionization	-interaction of functionins
-additivity assumption	-"in vitro"/"in vivo"
-hierarchial	-functional adaptation
-standardized/normative	-flexible/individualized

Research to date has yet to clearly suggest that either approach, reductionistic or dynamic, have an advantage in terms of rehabilitation outcome. Theoretically, these models do not have to be mutually exclusive. In the clinical world, most practitioners integrate both approaches to some extent. Nonetheless, these assumptions have significantly influenced research methodology in neuropsychological rehabilitation. The following review of literature provides examples of each approach to the rehabilitation of neuropsychological defects, and is not intended to represent the entirety of available research in neuropsychological rehabilitation.

Visual Spatial Disorders

Diller and Weinberg (7) and Diller and Gordon (8) have provided important findings regarding the treatment of visual spatial defects following right hemisphere brain damage in stroke patients. Defects in hemi-spatial inattention and visual scanning defects were treated with a very systematic and standardized regime, involving a hierarchial sequence of training modules. Patients were initially treated with tasks requiring them to attend to the left side of space and advance to more complex visual integrative tasks, involving scanning and spatial constructions. These investigators demonstrated significant improvements in treated versus non-treated subjects in visual spatial abilities, which also generalized to non-treated behaviors, such as reading.

A multi-modal approach to the treatment of visual spatial defects was described in a case report by Rao and Bieliauskas (9). These investigators treated a patient two and one-half years post right temporal lobectomy with perceptual training, self-instructional techniques and psychotherapy. Following treatment, the patient demonstrated significantly improved performance on neuropsychological tests, a resumption of leisure reading and driving, improved social skills and vocational activity. Which aspect of the treatment accounted for the improvements is unclear with this methodology, which is one certain limitation to a dynamic and multi-modal approach to rehabilitation. However, the potential to impact functional (in vivo) behaviors according to their reciprocity and interaction has been demonstrated through this case study.

Attention and Memory Disorders

Sohlberg and Mateer (10) treated four brain injured patients with a systematic attention training program constructed to address five different components of attention. These components of attention were derived from experimental research in cognitive psychology, and included focused, sustained, selective, alternating and divided attention. Remediation methods were derived for each of these components and the patients were treated from five to ten weeks. These investigators reported gains on non-treated neuropsychological tests of attention for all four patients. This approach emphasized targeting specific test deficits and providing analogue remediation based upon componential task analysis. Treatment gains were derived in terms of level of performance relative to

normative data for a criterion measure of attentional
functioning.

Comparison of treatment strategies for verbal memory
defects was performed by Gasparrini and Satz (11). These
investigators studied paired associate learning and recall
with thirty left hemisphere damaged subjects. When
comparing visual imagery to rote rehearsal strategies,
experimental subjects showed improvement with imagery only
on the task used for training. However, when experimental
subjects served as their own controls and where semantic
elaboration was compared with visual imagery, the visual
imagery strategies were found to be clearly superior to
semantic elaboration. The treatment intensity was quite
limited in the study and no analysis of individual
differences was offered.

Malec and Questad (12) used semantic elaboration,
visual imagery and teaching the patient to self-generate
questions about information to be remembered to treat a
brain injured subject for six weeks. Significant
increases were noted on neuropsychological measures of
memory functioning post-treatment. It should be noted
however that the patient was only twelve weeks post
injury, but the fact that improved neuropsychological
functioning was found for only memory functions suggested
that treatment outcome was not solely attributable to
spontaneous recovery. Gianutsos and Gianutsos (13) used an
eloquent and useful multiple baseline methodology to test
the effectiveness of semantic elaboration for word recall.
These investigators demonstrated that in some case the
therapeutic intervention was quite helpful in enhancing
word recall, but results were variable as a consequence of
emotional, age-related and the presence of other
neuropsychological defects.

These studies, among others, suggest that certain,
but sometimes equivocal, gains in neuropsychological

functions can be obtained with treatment. The rehabilitation of certain neuropsychological defects, such as memory, clearly in part relates to other individual factors. This reality may raise some questions about the appropriateness of remedial "packages" to treat certain classes of neuropsychological defects. Single case studies have generally utilized multi-modal approaches, whereas group studies have emphasized standardized treatment regimes. The research to date does not favor either what has been described as reductionistic or dynamic approaches to the treatment of neuropsychological defects. What is left quite unclear is the matter of who responds to what kind of treatment. The currently available research does not elucidate why one patient benefits from treatment and another, with a comparable severity of impairment in, for example, memory or attentional functions, does not.

RECOVERY OF FUNCTION AND NEUROPSYCHOLOGICAL REHABILITATION

As precursor and adjunct to rehabilitation efficacy research, the study of determinants of recovery have been the focus of recent research at the Center for Neuropsychological Rehabilitation (CNR). This section of the present work will address the assumptions and findings of a program of research being conducted at CNR designed to begin to address some of the questions previously raised.

The past research has largely focused on a particular neuropsychological function, such as attention or memory, as a generic defect following brain injury. One of the most difficult aspects of research in neuropsychological rehabilitation, however, is the significant heterogeneity of memory defects within and between diagnostic populations. Without controlling for or describing the heterogeneity within an experimental paradigm, there are likely limits on the generalizability of a given finding difficulties in duplicating findings. The other aspect of research in neuropsychological rehabilitation which makes efficacy studies complex is that many other personological, neuropsychological and environmental variables, among many others, may uniquely influence a given neuropsychological function, such as memory. Therefore, the scope of patient variables which may need to be studied grows exponentially. For these reasons, and given the state of knowledge in neuropsychological rehabilitation, the program of research being conducted at CNR has focused on individual determinants of recovery and qualitative differences in syndromes of impairment.

This line of research, considered a precursor to efficacy and outcome research, is for the moment focused on the traumatic brain injured patient, and is based on the following assumptions:

1) Complex psychological functions, which are represented diffusely or through multiple centers in the brain, are differentially effected through variability in the pathophysiology of the traumatic event;

2) As a consequence of pathophysiological variability, as well as other biological, psychological and environmental factors, complex psychological functions are disrupted in qualitatively unique ways;

3) These qualitative differences are relevant to the course of recovery of psychological functions, and as a consequence are relevant to how the patient should be treated.

Study 1-Pathophysiological Determinants of the Recovery of Attentional Disorders

Clinical observation suggested that there were important qualitative differences in the types of attentional disorders presented by patients with traumatic brain injury. Research by Van Zomeren and Deelman (14)

and Van Zomeren, Brouwer and Deelman (15) has suggested
that attentional defects following traumatic brain injury
(TBI) largely resolved within the first year post injury,
at least as measured with a reaction time paradigm. Our
hypotheses however were that while chronicity, or time
since injury, may be related to the degree of attentional
disturbance, different types of attentional disorders may
be characteristic of different recovery stages. We
further hypothesized that severity of injury, as measured
by length of coma, may be a determinant of severity and
type of attentional disorder. We further hypothesized
that variability in pathophysiological syndromes would
influence the severity and quality of attentional
disorder.

Seventy TBI subjects were considered for the study.
The mean age was thirty-two and the range was sixteen to
sixty-two. The subjects were classified in two ways: 1)
according to chronicity and 2) pathophysiological
syndromes (the reader is referred to Trexler and Zappala
(16) for details). Subjects considered for the study
presented with pathophysiological evidence of
predominantly either orbitofrontal, frontolateral or brain
stem-cerebellar pathophysiological syndromes. All
subjects were given a number of neuropsychological tests
of attentional functions, ranging from reaction times to
more complex mental flexibility and mental control. The
results can be summarized as:

1) No significant differences in either degree or
type of attentional disorder was found among patients with
varying severity or as a function of chronicity;

2) TBI patients classified as having predominantly a
more frontolateral injury had significantly more
impairment on measures of mental control and attention
shifting as compared with either the orbitofrontal or
brain stem-cerebellar groups; and

3) Speed of processing, regardless of task complexity, was more impaired in the brainstem-cerebellar group.

These findings supported the concept that defects in attentional disorders were not linear as a function of severity, at least as defined by length of coma. Rather, it was concluded that pathophysiological variability is in fact related to the quality of attentional defects. Future research is needed to determine if these different types of attentional disorders recover differently over time and whether or not different forms of neuropsychological rehabilitation positively influence that course of recovery.

Study 2-Recovery of Memory Defects following TBI

As in the case of attentional disorders, clinical observation suggested that the quality of memory defects following TBI were not homogeneous within the TBI population, nor was their course of recovery. Assuming some validity to these assumptions, neuropsychological rehabilitation of memory disorders would need to be driven by the determinants of this variability for each case.

In this study twenty-three TBI subjects who were evaluated and treated at CNR were included. Again, two methods of classifying the subjects were utilized. The first was a multifactorial severity classification schema was developed, based upon length of coma, period of retrograde an posttraumatic amnesia, time since injury and age. The total sample was divided into two severity groups based upon a bi-modal distribution of a composite severity index. These two groups were roughly characterized as "mild" and "severe" groups. The second classification scheme concerned pathophysiological syndrome, as was identical to that discussed in Study 1.

All subjects were evaluated with a number of memory tests, that included measures of immediate and delayed visual and verbal recall, recognition, verbal learning and susceptibility to interference, among others. Further, results from personality evaluation were included, as clinical observation suggested a relationship between emotional functioning and recovery of memory functions. Further, all subjects had been treated in the Day Treatment Program at CNR. Following a period of treatment, all subjects were again evaluated with all memory and personality measures. For a description of the treatment and details of the present study, the reader is referred to Trexler and Zappala (17). Results of this study will again be summarized:

1) Despite significant differences in severity between the mild and severe groups, no significant differences in memory or personality functioning were found pre-treatment;

2) The mild group showed significantly improved memory functioning over the treatment period, whereas the severe group failed to show any statistically significant gains;

3) Recovery of memory was found to be significantly correlated with the presence of positive acute neuroradiological findings, including presence of hematoma, brain stem contusion, among others;

4) Recovery of memory functions was not consistently correlated with any one of the severity variables, but poor recovery of memory was related to a higher incidence of frontolateral and brain stem-cerebellar damage;

5) Measures of ego strength were found to significantly and consistently correlate with recovery of memory functions, such that as ego strength improved over the treatment period so did memory functions; and

6) At six month follow-up, seventy-three percent of the mild group and thirty-five percent of the severe group had returned to work.

These findings suggest that while composite severity indices may be useful for research methods in classifying patients, their relevance for predicting recovery may be limited. Further, the results suggest that initial neuropsychological test findings may not be particularly useful in and of themselves and need to be considered in terms of other pathophysiological and neuroradiological findings. Finally, personological factors, such as ego strength, may have a direct relationship with recovery of neuropsychological function.

SUMMARY

A number of important clinical issues remain unaddressed as they relate to recovery and neuropsychological rehabilitation methodology. Certainly the herein described research does not fully answer relevant questions concerning attention and memory. Rather, and more importantly, these two studies characterize an approach to the study of individual psychological differences in a single diagnostic group as they relate to recovery and neuropsychological differences. Many other biological, personological, neuropsychological and environmental variables certainly influence course of recovery and neuropsychological rehabilitation methodology. The differential effects of variability in pathophysiology on the recovery of complex psychological processes requires additional research.

Other clinical issues related to recovery of psychological functioning and rehabilitation include the problem of defects in awareness and the relevance of pre-morbid and reactive personality disorders. Neurobehavioral and "pseudo-psychiatric" disorders have been receiving increasing attention in the literature as has new psychopharmacological approaches. All of these considerations relate to how patients recover from brain damage and, correspondingly, how they should be treated through neuropsychological rehabilitation.

REFERENCES

1. Trexler, L.E. In: Neuropsychological Treatment of Head Injury (Eds. A.-L. Christensen and D. W. Ellis), Martinus Nijhoff Publishers B.V., Boston, in press.
2. Trexler, L.E. In: Neuropsychological Rehabilitation (Eds. M.J. Meier, A.R. Benton and L. Diller), Churchill Livingstone, London, 1987, pp. 437-460.
3. Reitan, R.M. and Davison, L.A. (Eds.), Clinical Neuropsychology: Current Status and Applications, Winston and Sons, New York, 1974.
4. Luria, A.R., Higher Cortical Functions in Man, Basic Books, New York, 1966.
5. Christensen, A.-L., Luria's Neuropsychological Investigation: A Manual. Munksgaard, Copenhagen, 1975.
6. Basso, A., Capitani, E. and Vignolo, L.A. Archives of Neurology 36: 190-196, 1979.
7. Diller, L. and Weinberg, J. In: Advances in Neurology, Vol. 18 (Eds. E.A. Weinstein and R.P. Friedland), Raven Press, New York, 1977, pp. 63-82.
8. Diller, L. and Gordon, W.A. J. Consulting and Clinical Psych. 49: 822-834, 1981.
9. Rao, S.M. and Bieliauskas, L.A. J. Clinical Neuropsychology 5: 313-320, 1983.
10. Sohlberg, M.M. and Mateer, C.A. J. Clinical and Experimental Neuropsychology 9: 117-130, 1987.
11. Gasparrini, B. and Satz, P. J. Clinical Neuropsychology 1: 137-150, 1979.
12. Malec, J. and Questad, K. Archives of Physical Medicine and Rehabilitation 64: 436-438, 1983.
13. Gianutsos, R. and Gianutsos, J. J. Clinical Neuropsychology 1:17-136, 1979.
14. Van Zomeren, A.H. and Deelman, B.G. J. Neurology, Neurosurgery and Psychiatry 41: 452-457, 1978.
15. Van Zomeren, A.H., Brouwer, W.H. and Deelman, B.G. In: Closed Head Injury: Psychological, Social and Family Consequences (Ed. N.Brooks), Oxford University Press, New York, 1984, pp. 74-107.
16. Trexler, L.E. and Zappala, G., Brain and Cognition, IN PRESS.
17. Trexler, L.E.. and Zappala, G., Brain Injury, IN PRESS.

4

REHABILITATION IN TRAUMATIC BRAIN INJURY - OBSERVATIONS ON
THE CURRENT US SCENE

LEONARD DILLER

Rusk Institute of Rehabilitation Medicine,
University Medical Center, New York, NY 10016, U.S.A.

Dr. Howard Rusk, a major figure in the field of rehabilitation medicine in the United States, defined rehabilitation as
the third phase of medical care designed to deliver services to
accommodate the needs and optimize functioning in the physical,
psychological, vocational and social areas for the individual
with enduring impairments and disabilities due to disease or
trauma. Dr. Rusk's insight did not predicate a particular
technical or theoretical breakthrough or the development of a new
diagnostic technique or therapy. Rather,it was based on the idea
of organizing all the services needed to help the individual, in
a way to meet the convenience of the patient and enhance utilization. While this idea hardly seems novel now, it should be
recalled that in the United States it emerged at the time of
World War II. It revolutionized delivery of services to the
disabled in a way similar to the introduction of the supermarket.
The supermarket was not designed to create new products. It was
designed to make shopping more convenient for the consumer.
Services for the disabled after World War II, when compared with
services for the disabled before World War II, may be likened to
the differences between shopping in an old fashioned small
grocery and shopping in a modern supermarket. Rehabilitation and

supermarkets became major American exports after the War and have been adopted pretty much around the world.

Two interesting ideas are closely tied to this. First, consider the patient with spinal cord injury who served as a model consumer of rehabilitation services. The patient appeared at a rehabilitation setting with multiple problems including decubitus ulcers, urinary complications, limbs without sensation or motion, loss of bowel and bladder control, shock and grief over the loss of body image and functions, facing a future with no capacity for "normal" sex, difficulty in returning to work, or returning to a house which couldn't be accessed because of the steps. To this must be added problems faced by the family in dealing with the patient.

In this situation, with many coexisting problems, how does one know what to treat and in what order? In a sense the problem of blending the treatment mixes to meet such a wide array of needs was addressed by breaking the different services down into a series of tasks, which the individual could master in small steps to achieve competence and self esteem. An internal logic evolved where activities related to recovery, e.g., physical therapy for motor and sensory disturbance were followed by activities related to self care which preceded activities in the psychological, vocational, and social areas. The success of the system was related to a second feature. Namely the critical criteria for admission, progress, and discharge were based on the ability of the individual to achieve independence which was defined in terms of the ability to take care of daily needs to function at home or on a job. Activities of daily living (ADL) and job placement were the basic points of rehabilitation which cut across all physical disease and traumas. They were observable and public and could be understood by all. Patients could understand how goals were set and achieved. Dr. Rusk was able to paint simple and clear pictures of what would be achieved if the U.S.Congress supplied the necessary funds and the public

at large could easily rally around this argument. Dr. Rusk's
message was heard and well received so that rehabilitation became
very successful.

Interest in the rehabilitation issues of civilians with TBI
did not create a significant stir in the United States until the
middle 1970's. Perhaps the network of high speed highways played
a role in generating such interest. While individuals with TBI
managed to trickle through the United States rehabilitation
service delivery system, they now increased in numbers and needs.
They began to pose problems in terms of how the conventional
rehabilitation service delivery system could make adaptations to
meet the service needs of TBI. However, since the early 1980's a
veritable tide of research, service delivery and consumer
activities has been set into motion. These recent developments
have resulted in an explosion of clinical and research activities
at a rapid rate. As recently as ten years ago, it was possible
for a single person to have personal acquaintance with most TBI
programs and scientific writings pertinent to rehabilitation.
This is no longer the case.

The recent developments maybe tracked along three major
lines, (1) consumer interests, (2) research trends, and (3)
delivery of services.

Consumer Interests. Patient and family interests found
their expression in the National Head Injury Foundation (NHIF)
which was established in 1980; NHIF now lists 15,000 members and
350 support groups with 24 State associations. Begun as an
information network for families who were seeking services and
support, the Foundation has achieved great success in calling
attention to the problems of the TBI and help to guide policy.
In many states a simple count of the number of TBIs could not be
attained since TBI was not listed as a separate category and,
therefore, could not be tracked down by state and local agencies
who were delivering services to this population. The growth of

service delivery programs for TBIs was also fueled by changes in
payment schemes encouraging the development of fee for service
programs based on profits and separated from academic and
research settings. The NHIF identifies 500+ programs which state
that they are delivering services to individuals with TBI. The
quality and adequacy of these services are difficult to judge.

Research - Two major branches of the United States Government
have funded research targeted at TBI during the past five years.
These include the National Institute for Neurological and
Communicative Diseases, which is part of the National Institute
of Health and the National Institute of Disability and
Rehabilitation Research which is part of the Department of
Education. The NIH research is focussed on more basic research
questions and has sponsored studies on epidemiology, coma
recovery, technical improvements in diagnostic procedures and
neural regeneration. NIDRR research has followed several paths.
(1) Sponsoring individual studies emerging from different field
investigator initiatives, (2) developing Research and Training Centers (RTC) which coordinate several areas of research studies and
disseminate the findings to workers in rehabilitation. The
studies in the RTCs have been mandated to examine recovery of
language, motor, cognitive and personal recovery and to conduct
innovative interventions and methods of assessment. (3)
Developing major centers which will attempt to establish model
systems for services. These systems are supposed to deliver
services and track individual TBIs from the time of initial
admission to a hospital, through acute and subacute inpatient
medical care, to the home or eventual long term disposition. The
model system approach is designed to reduce long term secondary
complications in chronic disability by emphasizing early
interventions and quality and training of services throughout the
course of rehabilitation. (4) Studying effects of supported
employment. A major thrust in vocational rehabilitation is to
encourage placement of the disabled person in an actual work

setting with a job coach to monitor and supervise the patient and to serve as a facilitator with an employer for as long as is needed. This approach bypasses the traditional approaches to counseling and job tryouts in favor of in situ interventions. It fits a philosophy of cooperation with private industry. It is, of course, impossible to summarize outcomes in these various areas. Nevertheless, TBI has become a priority in sponsored research in rehabilitation and has received support at the more basic neuroscience level. The National Head Injury Foundation has made its considerable presence felt in directing public research funds into this area.

Service Delivery. Over the past 20 years the Commission on the Accreditation of Rehabilitation Facilities (CARF) has been established to set standards for the provision of rehabilitation services., These standards have been used for quality assurance for third party providers and governmental agencies which fund programs. CARF currently accredits nearly 6,000 programs conducted in close to 2000 facilities. In the past three years CARF has developed standards for accreditation of programs in TBI. There are two kinds of TBI programs: Acute care which is hospital based and post-acute care. Accredited TBI programs are categorical, i.e., they involve services delivered to a given type of patient exclusively or nearly exclusively. An inpatient program must have 10 beds set aside for TBI patients and must see a minimum of 30 patients per year. The program must include assessments and interventions for cognitive, perceptual, behavioral, communication and affective problems as well as social services, recreational, leisure, vocational, sexuality, and legal competence services. It must have a designated team with a consistent staff who will work with the same patient over time. Services to families are also necessary. Each CARF program is required to have a method developed to evaluate its results. Post-acute care programs include residential or day treatment, or vocational settings. They may be short-term or long-term or even used only for respite care. The program evaluations include outcome measure of level of independence, productivity and psychosocial adjustment.

There are currently 42 CARF accredited programs for TBI. The standards are premised on the idea that TBI patients need special, intensive services delivered by teams who specialize in working with these patients over time. It appears as if the current generation of professionals is arguing that TBI rehabilitation is different from the more general type of rehabilitation conducted with patients in a comprehensive medical rehabilitation program. The intensity and person power requirements for such a program make it more expansive than conventional comprehensive medical rehabilitation programs. In the language of our original supermarket metaphor, a TBI population requires a specialized gourmet counter or shop.

System Issues. The rapid growth of programs has resulted in a bewildering array of services ranging from private practitioners in different medical and allied health fields to state operated facilities. At least eight states have developed commissions to set up criteria for patient selection, staffing and standards for care. One major development has been the growth of for profit organizations, some of which, e.g., New Medico are establishing national networks. A parallel development spurred by the NHIF is that of Provider's Councils at the state level to develop criteria for programs. What is needed is a system of services.

A system of care for TBI would cover (1) services for patients from coma to the community, (2) would have to provide for different kinds of services appropriate to individual paths of recovery.

(See Table: "ELEMENTS OF A MODEL SYSTEM OF CARE FOR TBI")

ELEMENTS OF A MODEL SYSTEM OF CARE FOR TBI

Emergency Care
Acute Medical Intervention Procedures

Neurosurgery / Neurology

COMA — Patient Cannot Actively Participate

COMMUNITY
- **RESPITE / RECREATION** — Non-Intervention Model, Socialization
- **HOMECARE** — Case Management at Home
- **INDEPENDENT LIVING** — Self Directed Home Program

ACUTE REHABILITATION — Inpatient Restoration (3–4 mos.)

SUBACUTE REHABILITATION — IP/OP (6–24 mos.)

BEHAVIOR DISORDERS — Destructive Behaviors Continuum Controlled Settings

DAY TREATMENT — Outpatient
- **EDUCATIONAL** — Outpatient
- **VOCATIONAL** — Variety of Services Toward Work Goal

TRANSITIONAL LIVING — Non-Medical Compensation (4–18 mos.)

LIFELONG LIVING — Lifetime Support Residential

The elements of a comprehensive service delivery can handle
the flow of varieties of TBI from mild to severe. There are as
yet no data as to how many such systems actually exist. Nor are
there data that suggest such systems deliver better services or
deliver services more cheaply. But even a superficial
examination of the figure raises a number of issues: (1) the
services are more organized at points close to the onset than
they are organized at the community level. (2) The services are
organized around ongoing organizatorial structures rather than on
the basis of actual studies of natural recovery. One might argue
that treatment should occur at the most likely times for
recovery. Sarno, M., and her colleagues, (1) for example, have
shown that language recovery in a group of TBIs tends to spurt at
periods between 3 and 6 months, 12 and 24 months after onset. (3)
In contrast to the traditional approach which is organized around
the perspective of professionals working in hospitals or
vocational agencies, the model system approach is consumer driven
and reorients the thinking of policy makers and resource
providers in terms of where efforts should be directed. It also
serves to redirect the attention to   different sets of issues
where efforts should be directed. For example, what kinds of
services are needed in the chronic phase of disability, how
intensive should they be, how long should they last? A systems
approach should permit gathering of new kinds of useful
information to help guide service in the field .

Vocabulary For Assessment

In considering the rehabilitation of TBI from a systems
perspective we immediately run into a difficulty. How do we
define the patient, and what is the problem which is being
considered for treatment. It is obvious that the range of
presenting complaints in TBI will vary in terms of severity and
type. The problems will be influenced by the setting in which
they are presented. They are translated into different
vocabularies by specialists using different types of instruments

and procedures. Furthermore, the language of assessment must be understood by a variety of professional disciplines, third party payers and policy makers as well as consumers and their families. It is also clear that different programs and procedures vary in their range in trying to influence pathophysiological, behavioral, and social events. All of the participants in rehabilitation are part of the system making, the issue of accountability even more salient.

Let us consider a model adapted from the more general field of rehabilitation of people with disabilities. This model is based on the distinction originally proposed by Nagi (2) to help crystallize thinking about the disabled. Nagi distinguished between impairments, disabilities, and handicaps.

Impairments refer to loss of structures or functions. Impairments maybe limitations in cognitive as well as physical structures. Thus, limitations in intellectual competence to explain why a person cannot perform a skilled act maybe viewed as mental impairments. Cognitive impairments maybe presumed to account for a great deal of the behavioral difficulties manifested by TBIs.

Disabilities refer to restrictions in functional abilities due to impairments which limit independence. Limitations in carrying out the activities of daily living are disabilities. If a limitation in range of motion of the fingers is an indicator of impairment, an inability to hold a cup would be an indicator of disability. In contrast with measures of impairments, measures of disability have face validity or content validity. In considering cognitive impairments, while it is not obvious that response to a given test item indicates an individual is more intelligent, an item on a disability scale does indicate a person is more skilled in self care. It is reasonable to assume that the ability to hold a cup or perform any other skilled functional act, may be valid markers of level of independence.

Handicaps

Handicaps refer to limitations in the individual's carrying out normal activities in accordance with premorbid or normative expectancies. While impairments and disabilities reside in the individual, handicaps reside in the person, in the environment or in their interaction. Thus, a child with a physical disability maybe handicapped in attending school. However, should ramps be installed, an environmental change, the child can attend school. A disabled worker who cannot hold a job because of a disability might be able to work, if the circumstances of employment were changed. The distinction can be put in another way. Disabilities are measured by skills--what a person can do. Handicaps are measured by what a person actually does. Impairments and disabilities are evaluated on scales of competencies. Barriers for the physically disabled, are usually considered in physical or architectural terms. However, barriers might also be legal or social. While impairment, disability, and handicap are usually correlated, this need not be the case. For example, the quadriplegic in a motorized wheelchair may be severely impaired motorically. However, he/she may be quite capable of navigating the environment. Similarly disability and handicaps are usually associated but this need not be the case.

In considering handicaps, one important distinction can be made. One can speak of two levels of handicaps. At a gross level handicap can be dimensionalized in terms of statuses, i.e., activities which can account for a great deal of the variance in what we do. Categories such as working, living arrangements, health care utilization and overall self help scores would fit this dimension. At a more refined level, one can develop measures of frequency and duration of activities. Attempts to apply such measures to people with spinal cord injury, stroke and cancer suggest that people with disabilities tend to spend an inordinate amount of time in passive as "opposed" to "active" pursuits. They spend more time at home as opposed to away from home. They spend more time alone than they do in the company of other people (3). Lezak (4) has noted the pervasive problem of social isolation in TBI.

Consider for the moment a rehabilitation program which assesses itself. Conventional assessment is in terms of whether the person has the skills to be more independent. Many of the quality of life issues which reflect what people do with their lives and how they spend their time are bypassed in such conventional evaluations.

When we apply this model of thinking to TBIs, a number of points can be raised:

(1) An assessment methodology should include a statement of etiology and parameters of pathophysiology. It might be well to consider the term TBI as an aggregate of pathologies, much as one considers cancer as a descriptor of a number of diseases rather than as a single entity. TBI is currently subdivided in terms of severity of brain damage indexed by a number of markers such as level of coma, duration of post traumatic amnesia, and other neurologic signs (5). Contemporary studies track recovery in patients with different degrees of severity. Among current issues here are (a) individuals with mild TBI are said to show pathological behaviors (6). Yet more recent studies of Dikmen, McLean, Temkin, Wyler, (7) find that when a control group of friends are assessed, the difference from normal shrinks considerably. (b) While it is commonly assumed that patients tend to plateau in cognitive recovery, at one year, recent evidence suggest that this need not be the case (8). (c) Furthermore, while some patients improve, some even get worse. (9).

(2) Medical complications.

Medical complications often may arise during the course of inpatient medical rehabilitation as Kalisky, Morrison, Meyers and von Laufen (10) have shown. Studies conducted during the first year of recovery suggest that more than three-fourths of such patients have medical complications which have to be addressed (11). Furthermore, these complications are often undetected or not recorded on medical records which are sent to inpatient medical programs.

(3) Impairments.

The major efforts in the field have been to use neuropsychological tests to characterize the impairments after TBI. However, we currently do not have adequate tests for some of the major clinical observations in working with TBIs. These include (a) how does one measure "acceptance" of disability in TBI, (b) the loss of executive functions in TBI (ability to initiate, plan, monitor, and evaluate sequence of activities), and (c) capacity for emotional self regulation. Perhaps more importantly neuropsychological tests are generally matched against pathophysiological measures, e.g., severity of TBI, but too often they are not matched against disability and handicap measures. (12).

(4) Disability.

Measures of disability as manifested in well known ADL scales run into limitations. First failure in self care such as dressing or feeding in TBI may be due not to paralysis but to a neurophysiologic disturbance. The internal dynamics of the disability are not captured by conventional assessments. Nagele et al (13) have shown that in brushing the teeth, the TBI patient may fail because the task involves a series of steps beginning from unscrewing the cap of a toothpaste tube to returning the toothbrush. Failure is more likely a byproduct of a breakdown in skill routine than a motoric disturbance. Second measures of activities of daily living are motorically dependent. We lack measures of skills which are cognitively based. For example, psychometric measures of memory, perception and problem solving yield only a gross indication of what specific tasks are failed in daily life.

5) Handicaps.

A major problem of TBI pertains to employment. Here recent studies (14) show that a sample of more than half of people with moderate to severe head trauma and had been unable to find employment despite all of conventional rehabilitation approaches can be returned to competitive employment even when interventions began at an average of 30 months after onset. The vast majority were able to maintain employment on followup studies conducted periodically up to 3 years. However, problems in family living may still persist. These figures are very similar to those reported on earlier studies in Israel (15) and the United States (16).

The outcome data reported by Ben-Yishay et al (13), is based on experience with more than 100 patients who have been seen since 1978. The program which is designed for outpatients is based on a holistic model which is divided into two phases. The first phase combines cognitive remediation, interpersonal skill training and counseling, in the context of a therapeutic community. It is designed to engage the individual and family in a therapeutic alliance to recognize the limitations and disabilities due to brain damage, to engage in tasks which maybe below previous expectancies built up over many years and finally to accept goals and activities which can make work and family living possible. The second phase which consists of occupational trials is designed to involve the individual in simulated employment which can provide a setting to test behaviors acquired during the first phase.

While it is difficult to identify in an experimental way which elements of a complex treatment program are responsible for success. Nonetheless, in a series of studies conducted in the program it has been shown that (1) in predicting return to work, when one takes into account demographic, neurological, neuropsychological test results and ratings of acceptance, all contribute to successful prediction, with perhaps the largest variance contributed by the ratings of acceptance (Ben-Yishay et al, in preparation), (2) when one varies the treatment hours in the first phase of the program to emphasize cognitive interventions, those receiving more cognitive remediation showed greater gains on neuropsychological tests, while those receiving more social and interpersonal interventions showed greater gains in personality qualities such as increased self esteem and increased interpersonal skills. However, in terms of employment both groups showed the same results.

Conclusions

Three major points maybe noted. First, there has been a remarkable increase in service and research in the United States with regard to traumatic brain injury over the past five to ten years. The field appears to be evolving very rapidly so that it is difficult to foretell what the future will bring. Second, an analysis of domains of behavior which are critical in assessing outcomes in rehabilitation - impairments, disabilities, and handicaps suggests that traditional neuropsychological approaches must focus on disabilities and handicaps as well as impairments to be maximally effective and that conventional approaches in rehabilitation based on working with other groups of disabled people may miss critical elements of the sequelae of traumatic brain. Third, with an intervention program designed to address the multiple needs of the person with moderate/severe head trauma, it is possible not only to facilitate employment in the majority of people, but to improve cognitive and interpersonal functioning.

REFERENCES

1. Sarno, M.T., Buonaguro, A., and Levita, E., 1987. Aphasia in closed head injury and stroke. Aphasiology, 1, 331-338.

2. Nagi, S.Z., 1965. Some conceptual issues in disability and rehabilitation. In: M.B. Sussman (Ed) Sociology and Rehabilitation, Washington, D.C. American Sociological Association.

3. Gordon, W.A., Hibbard, M.R., Egelko, S., Diller, L., Shaver, M.S., Lieberman, A., and Ragnarsson, K., 1985. Perceptual remediation in patients with right brain damage. A comprehensive program. Archives of Physical Medicine and Rehabilitation, 66, 353-359.

4. Lezak, M.D., 1983. Neuropsychological assessment, (2nd ed) New York: Oxford University Press.

5. Levin, H.S., Benton, A.L., and Grossman, R.G., 1982. Neurobehavioral Consequences of Closed Head Injury. New York: Oxford University Press.

6. Rimel, R.W., Giordani, B., Barth, J.T., and Jane, J., 1983. Moderate head injury: completing the clinical spectrum of brain trauma. Neurosurgery, 11, 344-350.

7. Dikmen, S., McLean, A., Temkin, and Wyler, A.R., 1986. Neuropsychologic outcome at one month post injury,. Archives of Physical Medicine and Rehabilitation, 67, 507-513.

8. Dikmen, S., Reitan, R.M. and Temkin, N.R., 1983. Neuropsychological recovery in head injury. Archives of Neurology, 40, 333-338.

9. Kay, T., Ezrachi,m O. and Cavallo, M. 1986. Plateaus and consistencies: Long term neuropsychological changes following head trauma. In: Proceedings of the 94th Annual Convention of the American Psychological Association, p. 175.

10. Kalisky, Z., Morrison, D.P., Meyers, C.A. and Von Laufen, A. 1985. Medical problems encountered during rehabilitation of patients with head injury. Archives of Physical Medicine and Rehabilitation, 66, 25-30.

11. Diller, L. and Ben-Yishay, Y., 1983. Severe Head Trauma: A comprehensive approach to rehabilitation. Final Report, Washington, D.C. - National Institute of Handicapped Research, U.S. Department of Education.

12. Hart, T. and Hayden, M.E., 1986. The ecological validity of neuropsychological assessment and remediation. In: B.P. Uzzell and Y. Gross (Ed) Clinical Neuropsychology of Intervention. Boston: Martinus Nijhoff Publishing Co.

13. Nagele, D.A., 1986. Neuropsychological inference from a tooth-brushing task: A model for understanding deficits and making interventions. Archives of Physical Medicine and Rehabilitation, 66-68.

14. Ben-Yishay, Y., Silver, S.L., Piasetsky, E. and associates, 1987. Vocational outcomes after intensive holistic cognitive rehabilitation: Results of a seven year study. Journal of Head Trauma Rehabilitation, 1, 90-99.

15. Hoofien, D. and Ben-Yishay, Y., 1982. Neuropsychological therapeutic community rehabilitation of severely brain injured adults. In: E. Lahar (Ed) Psychological Research in Rehabilitation. Israel Ministry of Defense Publishing House, 87-99.

16. Prigatano, G. et al, 1985. Neuropsychological Rehabilitation After Brain Injury. Baltimore: The Johns Hopkins University Press.

5

FUTURE DIRECTIONS IN REHABILITATION OF BRAIN INJURED PEOPLE

BARBARA WILSON
University Rehabilitation Unit, Southampton General Hospital,
Southhampton SO9 4XY, England

Rehabilitation can be defined as a process whereby people who have been disabled by injury or disease regain their former abilities or, if full recovery is not possible, achieve their optimum physical, mental, social and vocational capacity. In either case the process should lead to eventual integration into an environment which is suited to the needs and capacities of each individual. If those of us working in rehabilitation are prepared to accept this definition then we must also recognise that almost all aspects of a patient's life fall within our province. For neuropsychologists, this means accepting the fact that brain damaged people will be helped more if their specific problems are located within the wider context of their affected lives. Brain damaged people have bodies that may need rehabilitating, they have families with whom they must relate, they may have employment which they hope to continue, and, when they return to the community outside the rehabilitation unit, they will need to co-exist with others. In order to facilitate such goals, neuropsychologists will have to work in close collaboration with other members of rehabilitation teams.

In the main, psychologists working in rehabilitation are equipped to work on the cognitive, emotional and behavioral problems of their patients, although some psychologists will also become involved in the treatment of motor and sensory disorders. It is accepted that psychologists can do nothing to influence primary brain damage, and that each brain damaged patient brings a unique personal history of experience and leaves behind a pre-morbid capacity, neither of which can be reached by psychologists. However, psychologists, along with other members of a rehabilitation team, can influence the way a patient reacts to or copes with brain damage;

they can modify the reactions of others to the brain injured; and, in a more general sense, they can lobby for resources to support their particular branch of rehabilitation.

When designing a rehabilitation programme within the afore-mentioned parameters, a rehabilitation team must consider the following factors: the patient's age (on the whole the younger the patient the better will be the response to rehabilitation); type of brain damage (non-progressive brain injury is usually easier to deal with than progressive, and similarly, focal lesions are easier to work with than diffuse lesions); the family and social network (a patient with strong familial support will be easier to treat than one with weak support); the employer (a patient is more likely to get back to work with a sympathetic employer than with an unsympathetic one); and pre-morbid I.Q. (a patient with a previously high I.Q. is likely to respond better to treatment than one with a previously low I.Q., although it is worth noting that this factor is itself subject to several variables that cause many exceptions).

Having provided a brief view of the area in which we work and the boundaries imposed by the nature of head injury itself, and the training, expertise and, to some extent, status of rehabilitation therapists, I intend in the rest of this chapter to consider some of the future directions we might take in the rehabilitation of brain damaged people. In the process I shall refer to several main themes based on the work currently being undertaken by myself and others in the South of England.

EARLY ASSESSMENT PROCEDURES

There is a considerable gap in our knowledge about the natural history of recovery from brain damage, particularly from traumatic brain injury. This imposes limitations on our ability to assess recovery, especially in regard to the functional and practical skills needed in order to cope with everyday life. The widely used Glasgow Coma Scale (1) has proved useful for measuring the level of consciousness in early head injured patients. Although there are several scales available for monitoring recovery after coma, and for classifying outcome after patients have emerged from coma, these have proved to be less useful. The best known are the Glasgow Outcome

Scale (2), the Disability Rating Scale (3), the Stover and Zerger
Scale (4), the Ranchos Los Amigos Scales, otherwise known as the
Levels of Cognitive Functioning Scales (5), and the Neurobehavioral
Rating Scale (6).

Perhaps the most widely used of these is the Glasgow Outcome
Scale which exists in a short (5 category) form and in two expanded
(8 and 10 category) forms. Apart from the Neurobehavioral Rating
Scale, the remaining scales consist of eight categories or items
which by themselves are too broad to be able to detect subtle changes
in recovery. In a pilot study, for example, we found that tactile
exploration of objects always preceded visual exploration. Thus the
latter would appear to represent an important stage in the recovery
process, yet none of the above mentioned scales assesses this aspect
of behavior.

Another drawback with the established scales is that they cross
several behavioral dimensions, for example, motor ability, cognitive
functioning and social awareness, so it is difficult to identify
improvement in any one area. Although improvement in head control
and improvement in communication can occur independently of each
other, the established scales would not be able to distinguish such
separate changes in behavior.

Because of the breadth of the limited number of categories in
the above mentioned scales, certain behaviors exhibited by recovering
patients may fit into more than one category so that fine gradations
of behavior are lost (7). The effect is to produce a distorted image
of reality which helps neither patient nor therapist.

Another severe limitation of these scales is that they <u>rate</u>
certain categories of behaviour rather than observe or measure them,
thus tending to rely upon subjective interpretations which may not
reflect the true level of behavior. For example, in the Disability
Rating Scale one item is concerned with employability and four
ratings are permitted (0 - 3), but one person's idea of employability
may be quite different from another's.

A final criticism of these scales relates to the fact that they
do not specify the sequence of recovery stages in sufficient detail.
For example, item 4 in the Glasgow Outcome Scale is defined as 'can
travel by public transport and work in a sheltered environment and

can therefore be independent insofar as daily life is concerned.'
But the question remains as to whether ability to travel on public
transport precedes, follows on, or always goes along with ability to
work in a sheltered environment?

Other existing methods for assessing head injured patients,
including those which involve measurement rather than rating, have
further sets of limitations. None of them provide a clear
relationship between performance on tests and performance in real
life. When everyday skills are assessed directly, as in the
'activities of daily living (ADL) skills' monitored by occupational
therapists, there is often no measurement of the reliability or
validity of the methods used to collect data or indeed the results
obtained. It has to be inferred that the component items of many ADL
and similar scales have been selected intuitively.

Even when items have been selected through a process of
systematic observation they may turn out to be inappropriate for use
with head injured patients. The Barthel Scale (described in Wade et
al (8) is probably the best established and most widely used ADL
scale but its limitations are substantial: it has been validated for
use with stroke, not head injured patients; and even more worrying is
the fact that patients can score normally on the Barthel but still
have deficits such as amnesia which prevent independent living.

Existing measures cannot be employed at all stages following
head injury. For example, most neuropsychological tests cannot be
used with people just emerging from coma. Diller (personal
communication) says that 27 per cent of the patients admitted to his
center in New York are untestable on all formal neuropsychological
assessment procedures.

Another limitation of existing tests is that their measurements
cannot be employed across the spectrum of varying degrees of
severity. Many tests cannot, for example, be given to patients with
severe motor, sensory or cognitive handicaps, although objective
measures of such handicaps are urgently required. Finally, existing
measurements have little or no predictive power regarding final outcome and thus they provide inadequate information for guiding or
designing treatment programmes.

It should be possible to design assessments that are free from the weaknesses listed above and that can be properly administered by professionally trained people such as psychologists, occupational therapists, physiotherapists, speech therapists, nurses and doctors. One way this may be achieved lies in the adaptation of some of the procedures used in the assessment of people with mental handicap. Many of these assessments are influenced by behavioral techniques: they tell us what a person _does_ rather than what a person _has_ (for example, "this man forgets people's names and cannot remember the date" rather than, "this man has amnesia"); they sample behavior in different situations and under different conditions; and they establish a direct relationship with treatment.

It is possible to combine a psychometric and behavioral approach within one assessment procedure. For example, the Rivermead Behavioural Memory Test (9) is administered and scored like any conventional psychological test, but instead of using experimental or artificial material, the tasks in the test are similar to those demanded for normal functioning in everyday life.

A procedure that has been developed as a teaching technique for the parents of pre-school children suffering from mental handicap is Portage. Named after a town in Wisconsin, Portage assesses subjects on five developmental scales: _motor, language, self-help, socialization_ and _cognition_. The items cover the range of 0 to 6 years. Gaps in functioning are pinpointed and there is a clear cut relationship between assessment and treatment. The treatment is centred around developmental gaps, one or two of which are selected for treatment each week. Specific objectives (ones that are almost certain to be achieved within the week) are set, and a treatment programme is worked out between the home adviser and the parents. Portage has already been used with brain damaged people, including severely head injured people who are too impaired for more conventional assessments (10). Therapists have been involved rather than parents. There are several advantages to a Portage approach: it is adaptable to a fairly wide range of ability levels; most of the items can be completed either by observation or interview with carers thus avoiding motivational problems or the need for parallel versions; and it looks at real life skills rather than performance on experimental material. Tasks employed by Portage can be included in a 'purpose-built' assessment of early head injuries emerging from coma. More adult oriented items can be selected from established assessments of adults with mental handicap (for example, Bereweeke (11) and the Hampshire Assessment for Living with Others (12). Using a developmental approach to measure recovery after head injury is not new (see, for instance, Eson (13), nor necessarily appropriate. However, the adaptation of this approach might reveal that recovery of certain functions follow the developmental pattern whereas others do not.

Bereweeke (an adult version of Portage) and HALO go beyond developmental stages and cover a wide range of skills required for everyday living. HALO also assesses how much help each testee requires in order to perform these skills. Thus by combining Portage, Bereweeke and HALO with some existing ADL tasks and behavioral rating scales, a comprehensive assessment can be developed to cover all stages of recovery and all degrees of severity following head injury. Furthermore, such an assessment would concentrate on practical skills, provide a finely graded record of change throughout recovery, and establish a clear link between assesment and treatment.

There are disadvantages in using these scales with traumatically brain injured people as many of the items are inappropriate for adults. Nevertheless, the experience gained from using this approach in the field of mental handicap can guide the development of assessment scales with people who sustain brain damage in adulthood.

Research in this area is currently being carried out in Southampton and at the end of our study we hope to answer a number of questions including the following: Is there a consistent pattern in the recovery of various functions (physical, cognitive, emotional etc.) or does this vary widely? If there is some consistency does it follow the developmental pattern or some other? To what extent can the nature and rate of early recovery provide clues to long-term prognosis? To what extent can this be systematized into a useable set of scales?

Items we are working on currently include the following categories of behavior, looked for in patients soon after they have emerged from coma.

Head Control

None	0
Attempts to lift head	1
Maintains head posture for 5 seconds	2
Lifts and maintains head posture for 1 minute	3
Lifts and maintains head posture more than 1 minute	4

Tactile Awareness

None	0
Moves in response to touch	1
Removes cloth from face	2
Tactile exploration – texture	3
Tactile exploration – form	4

Smiling

None	0
Apparently random	1
Smiles in response to close relatives	2
Smiles in response to nurse/therapist	3
Smiles appropriately to relatives/staff/patients	4

Method of Expression

None	0
Eye points	1
Uses facial expressions	2
Uses gesture	3
Uses mime (elaborated gesture)	4

Visual Awareness

None	0
Tracks and follows moving object 3 - 5 seconds	1
Explores picture visually	2
Looks at visitor when requested	3
Looks at stimulus on 3 consecutive occasions	4

EARLY TREATMENT

Early treatment programmes such as Coma Management (Sensory Stimulation) are widely practised in the United States and elsewhere. Although some of these programmes may turn out to be useful in promoting better or faster recovery, we are not in a position to give an answer to this question because the proper evaluations of such programmes have not taken place. It is essential that such evaluation is carried out to ensure that progress is made in rehabilitation. Sensory stimulation programmes typically involve the patient being stimulated in several different modalities for a few minutes several times a day. Auditory stimulation procedures, for example, might involve talking to the patient, explaining what has been happening, playing tapes made by family members, playing the patient's preferred music, and providing orientation information. Tactile stimulation might involve carrying out a range of passive movements exercises, frequent changing of position, gentle brushing or icing techniques, and providing the patient with experiences of various pressures and touches. Visual stimulation (which can of course take place only after the patient's eyes are open) might include presenting photographs of the family, favourite pop stars, and other personally relevant stimuli.

It is quite possible that such early stimulation will hasten recovery. However, it is also possible that we can do damage to the patient by stimulation during coma. Our knowledge is insufficient to support claims in favour of early stimulation, and until we carry out objective evaluations, we are perhaps following a dangerous line by merely giving reign to our intuitions. After all, a worthy hypothesis might suggest that the brain, whilst in a position of being 'switched off' during coma, is in fact reducing the demands made upon it thus giving itself a better chance of recovery. The assessment scales described earlier would be helpful in measuring response to treatment. If it transpires that the claims for systematic stimulation are indeed supported by the results from objective assessment and evaluation using such instruments, then we would be able to move forward more confidently.

It is not unreasonable to expect that learning can take place during coma. Boyle and Green (14) reported the use of operant procedures with comatose patients after they had worked with three patients who had been in coma for periods of six, ten and thirty eight months. The authors attempted to teach their patients to squeeze their eyes or make a movement to a verbal request by rewarding them with a fifteen second tape excerpt of favourite music. The patient who had been in coma for six months learned all three of the behaviors attempted whereas the remaining two learned to comply to only one of the behaviors.

WORKING MORE CLOSELY WITH OTHER DISCIPLINES
Although most people seem to agree with the idea of multi-disciplinary and inter-disciplinary team work there seems to be very little of it going on except for joint discussions and work that runs in parallel through departments. Yet it is possible to devise inter-disciplinary treatment which enables therapists from several disciplines to work together to design, supervise and assess programmes. At Rivermead Rehabilitation Center in Oxford, England, for example, a young woman with quadriplegia and dysarthria following brainstem encephalitis was taught by an inter-disciplinary team to carry out a variety of tasks to aid greater independence (10).

This young woman had developed brainstem encephalitis 18 months prior to treatment. She was consequently quadriplegic and severely dysarthric. A Portage programme was used to teach her a number of tasks to increase her independence. Her physiotherapist, occupational therapist and clinical psychologist met each week to select the overall goal, the sub-goals or tasks for the coming week, and to take baselines and supervise the observation and documentation that was required for recording progress. One of the first sub-goals was to teach the young woman to drink half a cup of tea

independently. During morning and afternoon tea breaks, when the
young woman was seated at a bench in the canteen, half a cup of tea
was placed in front of her, she was asked to reach for the tea and
drink it unaided. She was allowed to stop and start as often as
necessary, but had to be finished by the end of the break. It was
decided by the team that if she was unable to manage this task she
would be initially encouraged verbally, and if this failed she would
be supplied with a weighted cuff to her sleeve, and if this failed
her hand would be guided through the movement.

By the end of the first week the young woman was drinking a
half cup of tea but needed considerable verbal encouragement. The
task was continued for a second week, by which time she managed the
task without constant encouragement. Of course with this woman, as
with all patients, it was necessary to take into account her physical
limitations. We wanted to extend her capabilities but were
constrained by the nature of her handicap. For the most part we
appeared to be successful in striking this balance as she learned 8
out of the first 10 tasks (set at the rate of one each week)). The
tasks she failed were beyond her physical capacity so the failure was
due to the therapists' wrong choice of goals.

Another example taken from work at Rivermead involved teaching
a woman to co-operate in her physiotherapy regime (15) This young
woman sustained a severe head injury in a road accident when she was
22 years old. She was referred to clinical psychology because of her
fear of physiotherapy exercises. She refused to do most exercises
for more than one or two minutes at a time and her physiotherapist
became increasingly concerned about her. A programme was devised
whereby the patient was given feedback on the number of minutes she
spent on a particular exercise the previous day, encouraged to
increase that time, and rewarded with an exercise she liked doing if
she managed to beat her previous record. A multiple baseline across
behaviors design was used here with very encouraging results.

These two inter-disciplinary programmes, like many others
practised at Rivermead, involved a behavioral approach where an
appropriate task analysis was carried out, goals set, baselines
taken, a step-by-step teaching procedure implemented, and evaluation
carried out by means of detailed behavioral assessment and/or by a

single case experimental design. Such work usually springs from the discipline and skills of psychology, and indeed the impetus for such work came from the clinical psychologist. However, the selection of goals, the consideration of safety factors, knowledge of movement, swallowing mechanisms etc. were provided by the other therapists who formed part of the team, and who contributed to the design and supervision of the programmes at all stages.

WORKING WITH FAMILIES

Ultimately, members of the family of a brain injured person are going to be the major participants in the care of that person, and for this reason policies should be adopted which enable families to participate in certain areas of treatment from the outset. Much of the early sensory stimulation is normally undertaken by members of the family, and many behavioral management programmes encourage family participation. In a number of cognitive rehabilitation programmes the family will be involved in selecting goals, carrying out treatment strategies at home and so forth. Social workers typically spend a considerable amount of time with the family of a brain injured person. Physiotherapists are also likely to teach members of the family how to lift, transfer and manage difficult motor problems. It is also usual to find family support groups meeting in rehabilitation centers.

Nick Moffat, working in the South of England, has for some time been involved in running groups for the relatives of those elderly people with dementia who are still living in the community. For the first few groups Moffat interviewed the carers and asked them to complete a rating scale. The purpose was to discover what kinds of information to present at the group meetings. In the interview study the most commonly voiced concern was for information about dementia. This was followed by the need for information about how to cope with memory problems. The third most frequently reported request was for information about the problems other carers faced in looking after their elderly relatives with dementia. Fourth was information about how to cope with behavioral problems; fifth and sixth were requests for information about coping with anxiety and depression. These were followed by a concern for knowledge about the role of the occupation-

nal therapist. Then came the need for information about the
emotional states of other carers; ideas for activities for relatives,
and, finally, a need for knowledge about the role of the psycho-
geriatrician.

As well as the interview, the carers were asked by Moffat to
rank in order of importance the six areas to be considered by the
groups in their meetings. The order was as follows: information
about caring for their relatives; information about services
available; information about old age and dementia; access to
services; how to improve social contact; and, finally, how to care
for themselves.

As was pointed out at the beginning of this section, members of
a brain injured person's family will take ultimate responsibility for
the daily well-being of that person. It is also worth noting that
the care provided by a family is far less expensive than the care
that can be provided by the state or private health institutions.
For these reasons the health and well-being of family carers should
be a matter of concern to all of us working in rehabilitation. Thus
we await the outcome of the evaluation of Moffat's groups with
considerable interest.

SELF HELP AND SUPPORT GROUPS

One of the best known support groups in Britain is 'Headway',
the National Head Injuries Association. This organisation has been
in existence for several years and was set up to provide support for
the head injured and their families. It aims to heighten public
awareness of the special problems faced by head injured people and
their relatives. It has shown particular concern for the provision of
appropriate facilities for rehabilitation and short and long term
care. There are about 60 local Headway groups throughout Britain,
bringing together the head injured, their families, voluntary helpers
and professional workers. Similar organisations are to be found in
other parts of the world. In America, for example, the National Head
Injury Foundation acts as an advocate for head injured people and
their families.

Recently, the Amnesia Association (Amnass), has been launched
in Britain by Deborah Wearing and Barbara Wilson. Deborah Wearing is

the wife of a musician who developed Herpes Simplex Encephalitis in March, 1985. Formed in September, 1986, Amnass attempts to help relatives of memory impaired people under the age of 65 years. The association works for the relief of amnesic people and their relatives; it coordinates and initiates research into memory impairment, and disseminates information about amnesia to those directly affected, to those involved in diagnosis, and to various care agencies.

First and foremost, Amnass is an action group committed to the provision of appropriate long term care facilities for the memory impaired. It is hoped to establish a unit for long term residential and day care where the memory impaired can live in a comfortable and homely environment attended by specially trained staff. Amnass is also developing a network of regional support groups so carers and professionals working in the field of memory impairment can share resources and expertise. Further information about Amnass can be obtained from:

The Amnesia Association, 25 Prebend Gardens,
Chiswick, London W4 1TN, England.

Amnass publishes a newsletter called 'Recall' three times a year. There is also a scientific subcommittee of four psychologists and one psychiatrist which is working with a community medical officer to set up an epidemiological study in a particular health region to discover the incidence and prevalence of amnesic people.

Such self-help and support groups as those described above are likely to contribute much towards community rehabilitation programmes. This contribution will take many forms, including the development of research programmes, a widening of knowledge about brain injury, and a deepening of understanding of the problems faced by neurologically impaired people and their relatives. Above all, they will act as pressure groups to bring about improvements in the services offered to affected families.

LONG TERM CARE

In Britain little is available for brain injured people requiring rehabilitation. The provision of early care is haphazard and its presence depends in part on geographic location, whilst its

quality may depend on the policy of local hospitals and/or the
expertise and attitude of particular physicians. Many head injured
people are admitted to the care of orthpaedic surgeons because the
patients might happen to have broken limbs. Intermediate care (up
until one or two years post brain injury) is available to very few,
and specialist long term care for the brain injured is almost
non-existent - although a number of them will be found in units for
the mentally ill, the physically handicapped or the elderly infirm.
Such conditions are tolerated despite the fact that many brain
injured people can go on improving for several years. For example,
Wilson, White and McGill (16) describe a young man who was shot in
the head at the age of 23 years. The bullet entered the left occiput
and lodged in the left temporal area. Among other things, this man
became totally alexic. He was determined to learn to read again,
however, and sought help for this problem over a period of several
years. One serious but unsuccessful attempt to reteach him to read
was carried out three years after his injury. Two years later
another attempt was made using a different method. This time the
treatment was successful and in the space of a few months the young
man's reading ability changed from being totally untestable to an
ability to read at the level of a 12 year old. This stage was
reached five years after the accident and in the face of extreme
pessimism from most people involved in the man's care.

Help in the form of management counselling and family guidance
should be offered to brain injured people and their families long
after the injury has occurred. Such help was given to Ben, a man who
had a left hemisphere stroke at age the of 60 years. He suffered a
right hemiplegia and aphasia. He received speech therapy for several
months after his stroke but this stopped once he became angry and
frustrated during speech therapy sessions. Five years elapsed before
he was referred to the clinical psychology department to see if something could be done to improve the situation at home (which was
extremely fraught because of Ben's severe communication difficulties). All his language functions were badly impaired, he failed to
score on the Token Test (17), and scored at the level of a two and
a half year old on the Peabody Picture Vocabulary Test (18).
Obviously, his comprehension of single words was very poor. He

could make very few sounds and was never heard to utter a recognisable word. He was unable to write to dictation but could copy words and letters. His reading was also very limited, although he was able to put the days of the week and the months of the year in correct order when these were written on individual cards.

The speech therapists had tried to teach Ben a few signs four years earlier but again this was abandoned because of Ben's reluctance to attend speech therapy sessions. The clinical psychologist and speech therapist worked out a programme for Ben in which a visual communication system was employed. This was based on a system described by Gardner, Zurif, Berry and Baker (19) whereby Symbols were drawn on cards and were of two types, abstract and pictorial. Abstract signs were used for proper names and pictorial signs for objects and actions. Modelling was used to teach Ben the signs. This involved the psychologist showing the card to the speech therapist who then pointed to the appropriate object or person or carried out the required action. This procedure was reversed so that the psychologist pointed or acted. Finally, the card was shown to Ben who was then required to carry out the pointing or action. If he failed we modelled the procedure again. If he failed a second time, we guided him through the action.

The cards were introduced in the following order: Names (of patients, therapists, Ben's wife, and names of other staff members) which were matched to real people or photographs; common nouns (for example, 'cup', 'matches', 'television'), again matched to real objects photographs; verbs (such as 'pick up', 'open', 'shut', 'fall'); requests, in the form of pictures of things Ben might want, (for example, a cup of tea, an implement of one kind or another); feelings (such as 'tired', 'fed up', 'angry') usually in the form of pictures; times ('winter', 'Christmas', month of the year etc.); and adjectives (for example, 'big', 'round'), which were either drawn pictorially or abstractly.

Ben's wife was encouraged to use the cards at home and to draw new symbols as and when required. Before treatment one of the major problems for Ben's wife occured whenever it was necessary to change Ben's routine. Ben was unable to comprehend such changes before the visual symbol system was introduced, but afterwards he was able to understand and therefore accept such changes. He was also able, by using the cards, to refer to events which had happened in the past or were going to happen in the future. He looked through his cards frequently and often showed them to his therapists to remind them of something that had occurred previously.

Ben's comprehension was helped within a few weeks of starting the programme but he took much longer before he was able to use the cards himself in order to express his needs or feelings. After a year an investigation was carried out to determine whether pictures or abstract symbols were differentially easier to learn for different word classess. It was known that Ben could learn some abstract symbols as he learned the names of several staff members this way, but we were not sure whether pictures were easier in general or whether they were only easier for certain word classess. Ben learned all the nouns and adjectives taught using pictures and all but one of the verbs using pictures. With abstract symbols, however, he achieved a 72 per cent success rate with nouns, 44 per cent with verbs, and 39 per cent with adjectives. Thus, in general, it made sense to use pictures whenever possible.

Nobody would claim this system was as efficient as normal language functioning, but it did help Ben considerably. Furthermore, Ben's use of the cards reduced tension at home because a means of communication, however limited, had been established between his wife and himself.

CONCLUSIONS

In this chapter I have attempted to identify areas in rehabilitation which I think may be developed in the next few years. I have also discussed changes that some of us would like to see introduced even though they may not be on the present agenda. Better assessment procedures are urgently needed in the early stages following brain injury. We need to identify strengths and weaknesses in those areas which are important for everyday functioning. Potential benefits include better planning of rehabilitation services, better selection of treatment goals, and the provision of relevant information on problems and progress for patients, their relatives and members of staff.

As far as early treatment is concerned, coma management and sensory stimulation programmes are proliferating, but these must be objectively evaluated before we can pronounce on their true value.

The introduction of interdisciplinary treatment programmes may bring about improvements in rehabilitation of brain injured people, the ultimate goal being the full extension of potential for each patient.

Rehabilitation will improve if professionals working in the field establish better contacts with families of patients. It should be recognised that families have learned a lot about the management of brain injured people as a result of constant exposure to problems encountered in daily living, and that this knowledge can be put to good scientific use by therapists. In this way, families can be helped to cope with anxiety and stress, and learn how to modify certain behaviors.

Self-help and support groups are likely to increase in size and number in the near future. We can expect them to extend the help they can provide. They will also have an important role to play in exerting pressure on health authorities and other agencies to improve the amount and quality of rehabilitation services.

Finally, the importance of long term care has been stressed. It is never too late to teach an old dog new tricks, and we are beginning to recognise that rehabilitation does not stop one or two years post brain injury. Everybody working in brain injury, whether they are theorists, researchers, writers, teachers or therapists, will do well to remember that our final goal must be to improve the quality of life for those who have the misfortune to suffer such injury. Further connections must be made between lecture theatres and laboratories, between laboratories and rehabilitation centers, and between rehabilitation centers and the homes where the brain injured live out their daily lives.

REFERENCES

1. Teasdale, G. and Jennet, B. Lancet, 2: 81-84, 1974.
2. Jennet B. and Bond, M. Lancet, 1: 480-484, 1975.
3. Rappaport, M., Hall, K., Hopkins, K., Belleza, T. and Cope, N. Arch. Phys. Med. Rehab. 63: 118-123, 1982.

4. Stover, S.L. and Zeiger, H.E. Arch. Phys. Med. Rehab. <u>57</u>: 201-205,1976.
5. Hagen, C., Malkmus, D. and Durham, P. <u>In:</u> Rehabilitation of Head Injured Adults: Comprehensive Physical Management (Ed. C.A. Downey) Professional Staff Assoc. of Ranchos Los Amigos Hospital Inc. 1979.
6. Levin, H.S., High, W.M., Goethe, K.E., Sisson, R.A., Overall, J.E., Rhoades, H.M., Eisenberg, H.M., Kalisky, Z. and Gary, H.E. J. Neurol. Neurosurg. Psychiat. <u>50</u>: 183-193, 1987.
7. Gouvier, W.D., Blanton, P.D., Laporte, K.K. and Nepomuceno, C. Arch. Phys. Med. Rehab. <u>68</u>: 94-97, 1987.
8. Wade, D.T., Hewer, R.L., Skilbeck, C.E. and David, R.M. Stroke: A Critical Approach to Diagnosis, Treatment and Management. Chapman and Hall, London, 1985.
9. Wilson B.A., Cockburn, J. and Baddeley, A.D. The Rivermead Behavioural Memory Test. Thames Valley Test Co., 22 Bulmershe Rd., Reading, England, 1985.
10. Wilson B.A. International Rehab. Med. <u>7</u>: 6-8,1985
11. Felce, D., Jenkins, J., de Kock, U. and Mansell, J. The Bereweeke Skill-Teaching System: Assessment Checklist, NFER-Nelson, Windsor, 1983.
12. HALO: An Introduction to the Hampshire Assessment for Living with Others. Hampshire Spcial Services Dept., Winchester.
13. Eson, M.E., Yen, J.R. and Bourke R.J. J. Neurol. Neurosurg. Psychiat. <u>41</u>: 1036-1042, 1978.
14. Boyle, M.E. and Green, R.D. J. App. Behav. Anal. <u>16</u>: 3-12, 1983.
15. Wilson, B.A. and Powell, G. <u>In:</u> Handbook of Clinical Psychology (Eds. S. Lindsay and G. Powell), Gower Press, Aldershot, 1987.
16. Wilson, B.A., White, S. and McGill, P. Paper at Second World Congress on Dyslexia, Halkidiki, Greece, 1983.
17. De Renzi, E. and Vignolo, L.A. Brain, <u>85</u>: 665-679, 1962.
18. Dunn, L.M. Expanded Manual for the Peabody Picture Vocabulary Test, American Guidance Service, Circle Pines, 1965.
19. Gardner, H., Zurif, E.B., Berry, T. and Baker, E. Neuropsychologia, <u>18</u>: 275-292, 1976.

6

COST BENEFITS OF REHABILITATION PROGRAMS

DIANE V. BISTANY

General Reinsurance Corporation, Stamford, Connecticut, 06904, U.S.A.

I am honored to be chosen from among the many professionals in the insurance industry of the United States
of America to clarify why we are involved in the whole
process of "rehabilitation of brain damaged people."

In the United States, although our insurance coverage
and process for paying for injured and sick individuals
differs from other countries, I will attempt to show that
there are similarities and our concerns and involvement
should be parallel.

Prior to joining my present employer, General
Reinsurance Corporation, the largest in the United States
and the third largest in the world, I worked for many
years in a rehabilitation facility primarily treating
catastrophic injuries and illnesses, particularly spinal
cord and brain damage. At the time, very little was
known about long term management of brain injury cases.
Once the physical problems were treated these people
went home, to nursing homes, institutions, or maybe even
jail for those who exhibited criminal behavior.

Before beginning, I want to thank Dr. Anne-Lise Christensen for inviting me to participate in this conference with such distinguished speakers representing different countries. I want to also thank Dr. Lance Trexler for his recommending me to speak before you. I am honored to be chosen from among the many professionals in the insurance industry of the United States of America to clarify why we are involved in the whole process of "rehabilitation of brain damaged people."

In the United States, although our insurance coverage and process for paying for injured and sick individuals differs from other countries, I will attempt to show that there are similarities and our concerns and involvement should be parallel.

Prior to joining my present employer, General Reinsurance Corporation, the largest in the United States and the third largest in the world, I worked for many years in a rehabilitation facility primarily treating catastrophic injuries and illnesses, particularly spinal cord and brain damage. At the time, very little was known about long term management of brain injury cases. Once the physical problems were treated these people went home, to nursing homes, institutions, or maybe even jail for those who exhibited criminal behavior.

Fortunately, we have progressed far beyond that point. We know many can be helped and their quality of life improved. For this reason we are all present at this conference.

Medical and scientific disciplines have, and will continue to make advances; however, unless there is an application of these discoveries and knowledge, it is of little value.

The application of advances in brain injury treatment and rehabilitation management is extensive and costly.

In the United States we have two systems which provide financial coverage. First, for those who are medically indigent and/or of limited financial resources, there are state programs providing care. These programs are funded by tax dollars and have strict guidelines for eligibility and types of care covered.

The second is insurance which is purchased by individuals, as well as employers for their employees. This insurance can be accident and health, workers compensations, or third party liability. These insurances do not involve tax dollars but rather premiums paid by private individuals and businesses. The scope of coverage will vary depending on the limits purchased. For those injured in the course of their employment, the individual state workers' compensation board mandates specific medical and wage loss benefits, however, private businesses still pay the premiums.

In preparing for this presentation I learned about the type of medical benefits provided for individuals in Denmark and understand that medical and rehabilitation expenses are funded by tax dollars with the mechanism for payment through Denmark's social system as well as its 14 regions and 275 municipalities. Further, there is individual insurance which can be purchased as a safeguard in the event of a motor vehicle accident. However, these awards are limited and most often provide income for those unable to continue employment as a result of their accident rather than payment for medical and rehabilitation services.

I am told the Center for Rehabilitation of Brain Damage has been in existence for two years and is the first of its kind in Denmark to provide a comprehensive approach for the treatment of individuals who have suffered brain damage.

As it has evolved in the United States, the present state-of-the-art for treatment of post acute brain damage follows an educational model rather than a strict medical model.

As a result, deviation from traditional treatment has caused uncertainty and skepticism by those funding the care. In addition, funding sources are asked to pay for treatment on a long term basis. This treatment is viewed as more expensive than ongoing maintenance costs. But is it, really? I will discuss this further in a few minutes.

The point is, regardless whether it is the taxpayer or the general public paying for medical coverage, it is the responsibility of those of us administering the funds, by whatever means, to protect the financial investment that is being made. How is this done? I will elaborate on this point later.

At this time, I will discuss the rehabilitation process and the manner in which we manage it. The process focuses on the needs of the individuals treated.

We realize that unlike other types of catastrophic disabilities, people who have brain damage many times require various stages of treatment. These stages may involve different programs over an extended period of time. This time frame generally translates into years not months.

Between acute care and final outcome, which may or may not be independent living, there is what I call primary rehabilitation followed by specialized programs for; behavioral management and cognitve retraining, transitional living, long term living, and finally, permanent placement. The permanent placement may be independent living, home with family, home with an attendant or caretaker, or a group home. Between and following any of these a nursing home may be required.

The rehabilitation process should encompass not only the treatment required but the smooth transition from one stage to the other while maintaining a continuity of care. My experience has shown that disruption also means lost ground.

The rehabilitation process is costly, therefore programs and goals must remain realistic and achievable.

In my many years in rehabilitation, whether it be on the treatment side or the funding side, the dogma has been the team approach. Always preached but in many instances not practiced.

Rehabilitation programs identify the team as those treating, the one being treated, and the team leader. I view the team to be far more expanded from that concept. The team process must be expanded beyond the walls where the rehabilitation program is taking place.

I believe that rehabilitation cannot be truly successful without including as team members the family, the community, the potential employer, the one paying for services and the attorney, if one is involved. I am sure you will agree, that without everyone working in concert, the result will be less than optimal.

Do we truly understand the team process? Do we practice the team process? Or, do we each have our own agenda and our own goals which we may or may not make known?

If we are to be a team, then we must act as a team and recognize who the team members are and their individual roles.

Professionals providing treatment need individuals to treat. Individuals requiring rehabilitation need funds to pay for the treatment received. Those funding the treatment have a financial investment to protect. Unless we communicate effectively, understand the process, and the outcome to be achieved, we fall short of the responsibilities imposed upon us in the entire rehabilitation process.

Advances in medicine and rehabilitation is progressing to the point where more services are being provided. Individuals who suffer head trauma or are brain damaged are afforded better care as their total needs are attempted to be met.

New programs are adding a new dimension to the management and care of these individuals. Hopefully, we are improving quality of life as well as duration of life.

Whether it is the taxpayer or the general public who is paying for medical and rehabilitation care, we must understand what it is we are paying for. Accountability dictates the necessity for us to be involved and understand the needs of the disabled. Funding facilitates the rehabilitation process, but the type and quality of rehabilitation must be appropriate. We are investing in programs to lessen residual deficits, improve quality of life and to be cost effective. If we do not become involved, how can we understand what we do not know?

In the United States, a segment of the insurance industry began taking an active role in rehabilitation and medical management many years ago.

We learned quickly that the results not only were good business but also very humanitarian for those individuals being served. Most importantly, we also learned that quality care is also cost effective.

However, because there are various forms of insurance in the United States, the process of active involvement in rehabilitation is not the same throughout the industry. A segment of the industry, particularly, that providing accident and health coverage is just beginning to understand the benefits of taking an active role in medical and rehabilitation management.

There is now a realization by companies providing all forms of insurance, that services which are provided at nontraditional treatment centers can result in the saving of large amounts of money on a case-by-case basis.

In brain damage treatment alone, the sophistication of medicine is saving people who previously died. Those surviving are being kept alive, often for a normal life span.

Regardless of who we are or what we do, we are faced with an increasing population of disabled individuals who require treatment, rehabilitation and ongoing management. We have also learned that for brain damaged individuals the recovery process goes on for several years. Proper care and management enhances and many times, accelerates recovery, and improvement while minimizing deficits.

If we provide the appropriate treatment and lessen the residual deficits, we also lessen the costs. Appropriate is a key work, because inappropriate, unnessary, or prolonged treatment not only is less than worthwhile but it is expensive in terms of effort and money. (Case studies are presented showing cost and treatment benefits.)

CASE STUDY

B.A. -   23 year old married male with 2 year old son.
           Worked as laborer.
           Struck by car April 17, 1982

Injuries: right subarachnoid hemorrhage
           occipital skull fracture
           unresponsive for 40 minutes

Acute and primary rehabilitation care - 6 weeks
Discharged home with parents - wife left and filed
for divorce. Attempted out-patient therapy unsuccessful.

Problems: confused, lethargic, cognitive and judgement
           difficulties.

Specialized Program: April 6, 1983 - December 15, 1983

Results: Living alone and working in factory.
           No further costs anticipated.

Costs: Acute care and attempted rehabilitation:
           $30,000 - $DK 201,000

Specialized Program: $90,000/$DK 603,000

Without specialized program would require supervised
living and sheltered employment.

Projected Costs Without Program:

           Annual: $24,000/$DK 160,800
           Lifetime (49 yrs.): $1,176,000/$DK 7,879,200

CASE STUDY

TW –   32 year old single male
             logging accident: January 30, 1985

Injuries: right deep frontal intracerebral hematoma
             left frontal temporal hematoma
             right pneumothorax, fractures right distal
             femur, scapula, C6-7

Early Treatment:
             Shunt and ventilator
             On 2/13/85 - opened eyes

Phases of Treatment:

             1. Local General Hospital - 6 weeks
             2. Major Neuro-Trauma Unit - 14 weeks
             3. Extended Care Facility - 4 weeks
             4. Primary (acute) Rehab Facility - 10 weeks
             5. Specialized Program - 44 weeks
             6. Home Program - 12 weeks

Total Costs of Treatment: $489,000/$DK 3,423,000

Result: Living alone, ambulatory without aides.
             Working as janitor part-time earning
             $1.65/$DK 11.06 an hour. Has a companion 24
             hours a week.

Projected lifetime Medical Costs:

             Annual: $12,500/$DK 83,750
             Lifetime (34 yrs.): $425,000/$DK 2,847,500

Without Specialized brain damage program:

             Annual: $48,000/$DK 321,600
             Lifetime (34 yrs.) $1,632,000/$DK 10,934,400

CASE STUDY

E.A. -   20 year old single male - factory worker -
          10th grade education
          Auto accident - April 19, 1985

Injuries:
          Closed head injury - in coma - 4-5 weeks
          Developed seizures October 25, 1985

Acute Care: 8 weeks - $70,000/$DK 469,000

Specialized Rehab.Program: 16 weeks - $90,000/$DK 603,000

Result: Initially returned to work in gasoline station -
         now a clerk in food store. Will require minimal
         medical follow-up annually due to seizures.

Projected Lifetime Medical Costs - 51 years:

          Annual: $500/$DK 3,350
          Lifetime: $170,850/$DK 525,500

Without specialized program would receive $7,020/$DK 47,034
a year workers compensation. Projected payments for life - 51
years: $358,020/$DK2,398,734

All of us who are involved in this rehabilitation rocess are accountable, whether it is those who treat, those being treated, or those who pay.

Unless we work together, how can we determine what is needed? How it should be provided? And the outcome? Only through ongoing dialogue and a close working relationship can we understand and determine what is appropriate for each case.

We have found that the active role of the insurance industry in the United States has encouraged rehabilitation facilities and specialized programs to look at their own accountability and improve their expertise in order to maintain a high degree of quality care.

What do I mean by active involvement on the part of funding sources? I mean that we must learn and understand the medical and rehabilitation needs of individuals requiring care. We must stay abreast of and learn of new research efforts and treatment in rehabilitation. We must evaluate and re-evaluate facilities and professionals providing care. We must inform and educate rehabilitation professionals as to our needs, concerns, and goals. And, most importantly, we must recognize that good rehabilitation and medical care improves the quality of life and reduces the financial exposure on a long term basis.

It behooves all concerned to become involved in cases as early as possible, while establishing a positive rapport and creating an atmosphere of working together to achieve good results. This is important in all catastrophic cases but, particularly so when working with brain damaged individuals. The nature of this disability crosses over an individual's entire inner being - - physical, intellectual, cognitive, emotional and psychological. It is a complex and devastating problem not only for the disabled individual but also the family.

We are aware of the tremendous need and expense in dealing with the brain damaged. Much has been accomplished in the last ten or fifteen years in terms of rehabilitation and improved results. However, I do not believe we are there yet. I do believe that we are at a point where we need to examine - what it is we are doing, how we are doing it, and why are we doing it.

This is going to take the cooperative efforts of the head injured, families, rehabilitation programs, funding sources, the insurance industry and the communities. It is a shared effort and should be approached in like manner.

Funding sources and the insurance industry must work with the various rehabilitation programs providing care in order to know the services provided, the expertise of those providing it, as well as the results they achieve.

There has been a good beginning. However, I feel it is only a beginning, and continued effort has to be a cooperative one.

Regardless whether we are in Denmark, the United States or other countries, we have a common problem. Our experience and new knowledge must cross waters if we are to be truly successful and serve mankind. Our expertise will be enhanced by continued meetings such as this. Our goals and hopes are one and the same - help those with brain damage to enjoy life to the fullest within the limits of their residual deficits.

7

PANEL DISCUSSION OF REHABILITATION

BARBARA P. UZZELL and ANNE-LISE CHRISTENSEN

UZZELL: Some concepts presented during this Conference include the recognition that: 1) theories about plasticity encompass individual differences in response to changes or demands within a particular context; 2) the effects of psychopharmacological agents are different for brain damaged and non-brain damaged individuals; 3) outcomes of cognitive rehabilitation are different for mild and severe head trauma; 4) 27% of the brain damaged population is not testable; and 5) recovery patterns among brain damaged individuals are inconsistent. However, rehabilitation of specialized programs have been shown to be cost-effective.

In view of the preponderance of variability among individuals seeking rehabilitation services, I want to ask each panel member to comment on whether he or she thinks every brain damaged patient should be rehabilitated.

DILLER: That is an extremely difficult question to answer. I certainly would think that a trial at rehabilitation would be appropriate. I have been involved in prediction studies of outcome with many different kinds of subpopulations in rehabilitation. If your prediction is too narrow you may be less accurate, and on that basis be denying someone an opportunity for rehabilitation.

WILSON: I certainly think that rehabilitation should be available for every brain damaged person. If we take the philosophy that is present in the field of mental handicap, the argument is that if the patients do not learn, it is because we have not found the right ways to treat them. Often, in neuropsychology, the philosophy seems to be, for example, if a specific patient cannot learn it is because he may have a lesion in the hypothalamus. If we take the view from the mental handicap workers, we can take the onus upon ourselves and find a way to teach the patients. Obviously, we cannot get people back to normal, and we cannot always get them back to work, but we can always make things better than they currently are. If we see rehabilitation as problemsolving, and set goals right, and say "how can we get this person's everyday life better than it is now ?" then that is rehabilitation, as I see it. We can certainly do that for every individual.

COPE: I would like to second Dr. Diller's point about the dangers of prediction. I personally have been tremendously surprised at times at the response of certain patients that I would have felt were virtually irrecoverable. They were making very dramatic gains, even to the point of resuming professional level life and activity. We should have a balanced attitude towards the intensity of rehabilitation in various periods. Everyone should have the opportunity to get rehabilitation.

BIERING-SØRENSEN: I like the viewpoint that everybody should be rehabilitated. But the extent of rehabilitation is a much more difficult issue today. Currently in Denmark, brain damaged people get a rehabilitation of physical deficits, but for most, neuropsychological rehabilitation is lacking.

TREXLER: The goals and expectations which should determine the services are very complex. Providing services to the patient who is 20 years post-injury with a severe persisting post-traumatic amnesia obviously has different goals and expectations than a

patient who is two weeks post-injury. In that same
regard, we often use the terms: mild, moderate, and
severe injuries, where the goals and expectations are
different. However, the question arises as to the
definition of mild, moderate, or severe. I have certainly seen patients that had, relative to others, mild
or no motor symptomatology, who presented severe neurobehavioral defects and significant personality changes,
which ultimately were at least as disruptive to their
reintegration. So the question becomes, rehabilitation
for what? The other question that has developed is what
are we rehabilitating? Often we are not providing a
specific restoration of some deficit, but facilitating
the utilization of resources. What emotional resources
are available within the family network? What resources are available in the environment at large (i. e.,
a cooperative employer makes a big difference). Rehabilitation certainly depends on the resource side of the
equation.

BISTANY: I want to look at this issue from a little
different perspective. Anyone who has suffered a
tremendous injury with significant deficit needs the
opportunity to be evaluated in terms of the potential
for rehabilitation, immediately or later. The rehabilitation team can assist in determining what is appropriate for that individual, and for the family and
all involved in the individual with the injury.

ASTRUP: As a neurosurgeon who sees clients in the acute
phase of the disease and who participates in the
activities of the Center of Rehabilitation of Brain
Damage, I am not at all convinced that the limited
capacity and resources are being utilized effectively.
The problem of selecting the right patients is not yet
solved. This raises the next problems: how do we
evaluate what is being done? which patients will
benefit from it?

CHRISTENSEN: Stages of recovery after trauma need to be considered. It is very important that patients in the first phase receive not only physical and medical, but also crisis intervention and neuropsychological treatment as well. The outcome of this treatment may determine the further rehabilitation course.

STEIN: This is not really a fair question to ask to someone who is not involved in rehabilitation directly, but in basic research. The question is primarily political, and secondarily economic. The will of the people of each country will influence the decision. The key question is really an evaluation of programs. The evidence from the experimental laboratories demonstrates that the sooner you begin pharmacological and other manipulation, the more effective is the treatment. Windows of opportunity for current, that is pharmacological treatments, are relatively small. The longer you wait, the less likely you will be successful.

UZZELL: Would any member of the audience like to comment on the question of whether everyone should be rehabilitated?

FINSET: Certainly, I agree that prediction criteria are imperfect, and may be dangerous. In my Head Injury Rehabilitation Unit in Norway, however, we get many more referrals than can be managed. Some kind of prediction or selection criteria are needed.

RAFAELSEN: I challenge the meaningfulness of the question with our present knowledge. A parallel may be drawn with tonsillectomies. How many tonsillectomies over the last 100 years were performed without a control study, until ten years ago when Blue Cross/Blue Shield denied payment? Suddenly, a good large collaborative study developed. How many good multi-center studies on the effects of rehabilitation exist that meet stringent scientific criteria?

TREXLER: Actually the question goes very much to the heart of the matter. There is no question that rehabilitation, particularly of traumatic brain injury, is quite labor-intensive and expensive. Certainly, if techniques are ineffective, other uses can be found for our resources. If, for example, we look at the cost to maintain a brain injured individual, there are some very straight forward measures that can show the cost-benefit in teaching skills of independence to non-ambulatory, or non-self-feeding patients.

ASTRUP: As a comment to Professor Rafaelsen, over the years, I have realized that some problems cannot be solved by controlled studies. Within the field of head injury, it is very difficult to make uniform groups due to matching of demographic variables. I would like to ask a direct question to Diane Bistany about what is the evidence that has convinced the insurance companies that rehabilitation pays?

BISTANY: Each case has to be evaluated on some merit. Unfortunately, sufficient data do not exist, which indicate what proportion of the population of head injured will benefit more than others. The insurance industry has found that planning for individuals has benefitted from relationships with reliable and trust-worthy rehabilitation programs.

BIERING-SØRENSEN: Rehabilitation is important. However, we need consensus of items considered for core investigations utilized by all research rehabilitation projects.

WILSON: To pose the question: does rehabilitation work, is like asking: does medicine work? It is imprecise. Many questions cannot be answered using the traditional research designs, and that is why single-case experimental designs are useful. The group design reported in group percentage and means, do not tell us what to do with the individual patient. The multi-baseline designs

are not just single case studies, they are experiments
that enable us to discriminate between intervention
strategy, and natural recovery.

DILLER: An evaluation of a program is different from
case management evaluation. Both have their place and
are accountable.

RAFAELSEN: The representative from the insurance
company seems to be the only one who is convinced by
the evidence that rehabilitation works. Rehabilitation
is not easy, it is difficult, but we should be optimistic and not say this is another impossible task we
have before us.

STEIN: If rehabilitation was a pill that you could
swallow, then you would have much more effective
control over the situation. When a new drug is developed in the United States, it costs about 100 million
dollars to bring that drug to market. Most of that
money is spent on research and development and testing,
because the Food and Drug Administration has specific
guidelines that must be met in testing a drug. Unfortunately, or fortunately for the rehabilitation field,
the majority of people feel that as long as it does not
hurt, and it may help, there are really no controls
required.

UZZELL: Would a Panel Member want to comment on items
to be included in predictive or in evaluation criteria?

TREXLER: I think it depends on what we are trying to
project. Because, after treating a number of people,
the reason that I admit one person to service is
different from the reason to admit another. So I think
one has to be clear about what you are trying to do.
The individual differences in the pathophysiology of
the illness, as well as premorbid personality characteristics, are some core items.

ASTRUP: Spontaneous recovery, in my opinion, is one big
methodological problem, when rehabilitation is started

early. If we need to disassociate the effects of
natural recovery from environmental manipulation for
experimental reasons, then some way should be found.
STEIN: All the evidence shows that the earlier an
intervention is made, the better the recovery. To
withhold any kind of treatment until the spontaneous
recovery is evaluated is absolutely irresponsible. I
would sue any physician that openly proposed that kind
of experiment.
ZEINER: There is a developmental perspective to treatment, since rehabilitation is clinically a very young
phenomenon. Some kind of fruition or development should
be reached before testing the efficacy of it.
DILLER: The most urgent problem in the field is the
development of an index to demonstrate that there is
efficacy in the treatment approach. We have to continue
to explore the techniques because we do not have a good
scientific base for cognitive remediations and interventions.
WILSON: If you are going to predict, you still need
outcome measures to see if predictions have come true.
UZZELL: Would the Panel Members comment on the specific
methods for rehabilitation as insiders and outsiders to
the Danish system?
CHRISTENSEN: The patients in Denmark are mainly treated
with physical therapy in medical departments. They
continue to reside in a hospital, depending upon the
severity of the case. When the patient has finished
with treatment, the possibilities for further professional assistance are very limited. Three years ago,
the opening of the Center of Rehabilitation of Brain
Damage was made possible. Located in a university
setting, we can only have patients who are ambulatory,
and at least one year after onset of brain damage. In
the beginning the patients referred were most often
patients who had bleak possibilities of good rehabi-

litation outcome, but strong supportive families.

DILLER: We have a problem when patients are discharged from a hospital, without private insurance. The only resource to pay for treatment is our vocational treatment system. The people who do not meet the criteria for vocational concerns are not entitled to rehabilitation assistance.

CHRISTENSEN: What has been characteristic of the Danish system is no belief that functional recovery can be enhanced through neuropsychological rehabilitation. The main purpose of this conference is to provide new information about ways and means for successful rehabilitation.

ASTRUP: Help for complex orthopedic injuries in Denmark is excellent and comprehensive. For minor head injury there is no safety net.

UZZELL: There seems to be a lack of information for the mild head injured, as well as, severe head injured in all systems internationally. Families and professionals need guidance. Is there another method for evaluating rehabilitation?

RISBERG: Preliminary evidence suggests that mapping of cerebral blood flow shows changes in the functional state of the brain after therapy.

CHRISTENSEN: Our preliminary experiments with cerebral blood flow techniques even seem to be able to suggest methods for our rehabilitation procedures.

RISBERG: When looking at the data from the first eight subjects receiving rehabilitation at the Center of Brain Damage, we found they were so very different that we had to treat the data as single-case observations. If we do averaging, a lot of information for treating these patients is lost.

SNORRASON: I want to draw your attention to another technique, the topographical analysis system, which has been in clinical use at the Municipal Hospital of

Reykjavik, Iceland, for the past three years. It is a noninvasive method to evaluate the functional state of the cerebral cortex, but it is still at an experimental stage. Preliminary results seem to indicate a potential use of this technique in rehabilitation.

UZZELL: These developments suggest that we are just beginning to see the tip of the iceberg, as far as the use of these specialized neurophysiological techniques within a rehabilitation setting are concerned.

ØBERG: The focus needs to be on whether retraining, compensation or substitution is taking place. Improvement of our methods of assessment of these techniques is also necessary.

ELLIS: How can we assess neuropsychological evaluations better?

DILLER: Neuropsychological assessment and remediation is only one component of a much broader problem in rehabilitation. Rehabilitation is much more multidimensional. There are many more fine graduations of behavior which go far beyond normal assessment procedures. These have ecologic relevance for people's behavior and daily activity.

WILSON: In designing treatment programs both neuropsychological and behavioral assessments are needed. Behavior assessments are very similar to our ecological measures, and the neuropsychological evaluations reflect intellectual level, cognitive strengths and weaknesses. But it does not really give us information about everyday problems.

TREXLER: If the purpose of neuropsychological examination is to document deficits, then certainly the examination will be of limited value. However, if you want to ask the question: under what conditions does a patient's performance deteriorate, and under what conditions does it optimize, then a dynamic and a clinical exchange with the patient is required. The

objectives and goals determine what is the neuropsychological examination.

UZZELL: Following traumatic injury, the aggressive and
violent behaviors sometimes appear during recovery. In
Denmark violent and aggressive patients may not be seen
as often as in other countries. Would a Panel Member
please comment on the observed incidences of violent
and aggressive behavior among patients in other countries.

COPE: It may be that some of the programs here in
Denmark are seeing a preselected variety of patients
with a certain level of recovery. Patients who do not
have a certain level of recovery, may not be referred.
Therefore, the people who are not seeing these violent
patients, in fact, may only be seeing a segment. The
alternative view is that there are different techniques
and expectations for rehabilitating patients in Denmark
and the United States; one view perhaps less authori-
tarian, more indulgent, and more understanding of the
individual personality characteristics of the patient.

THOMSEN: I think we do see the aggressive patient in
Denmark, but we also see patients with sexual problems
who need treatment.

COPE: Since sexually deviant behavior has very poor
tolerance in our society as a whole, these patients are
often institutionalized. Three types of sexual problems
have been identified. One is the young brain injured
female who has a problem with sexual behavior in terms
of disinhibition. A second type is a young brain
injured male with the same problem. The third type is
an aggressive young male who becomes violent because of
a presumable association of sexual drive with frustra-
tion. The first two types would normally require
straightforward learning behavioral rehabilitation
techniques. The third type, however, does not respond
to behavioral techniques. Medroxyprogesterone, an anti-

testosterone agent, has produced dramatic responses and
reduction of both sexual drive and aggression in these
latter patients.

UZZELL: It is interesting that cross-cultural differences in rehabilitation are appearing.

Concluding this conference without resolution of
issues and concerns is not easy. The comments made
during the discussion have not always provided concrete
answers. Ideas and thoughts of importance for rehabilitation specialists everywhere have been expressed.
The cost-effectiveness of rehabilitation attests to its
continuation for brain damaged individuals and society.

8

PROGRAM FOR REHABILITATION OF BRAIN DAMAGE IN DENMARK

ANNE-LISE CHRISTENSEN, MUGGE PINNER and NICOLE K. ROSENBERG

Rehabilitation in Denmark has until recently
primarily been undertaken as Rehabilitation Medicine.
The main treatment offered to patients with central
nervous system disturbances has been physiatry and
occupational therapy. The physical treatment has been
efficient, but belief in radical changes or improvement
has been lacking. Rest has been considered the basis
for recovery. The prevailing theory has been that since
neurons in the central nervous system do not regener-
ate, the loss of damaged tissue is irreversible. If
improvement is possible, it will occur spontaneously
within the first year. Consequently, the number of
rehabilitation beds for the brain damaged population
has been rather few, and the possibilities for treatment sparse.

The increase in traumatic accidents during 1960 -
1970 together with improved neurosurgical techniques
have created a growing need for improved treatment and
caretaking of the brain injured survivors. Furthermore,
experiences and research in Denmark (1) have shown that
the most common long-lasting problems of the brain
injured patients are psychological, emotional and
behavioral.

Due to a grant from the Egmont Foundation, the
Center for Rehabilitation of Brain Damage was established
as a private foundation at the University of Copenhagen
on March 1, 1985. The grant was given for a three-year
period, where course and outcome were meant to il-

luminate the need for psychological treatment of this group of patients.

The main purpose of the Center is to offer treatment within the areas of cognition and social adaptation. The program treatment is designed to promote recovery of function to an extent that, in the best of cases, the patients may be able to return to work. Full time or part-time work, or work in so-called "protected jobs" are potential solutions. In the most serious cases an attempt is made to avoid placement in nursing homes and to enable patients to live with their families or in their own home.

The Center is headed by a Director, who is a neuropsychologist. The staff includes at present two neuropsychologists, three clinical psychologists, one psychology intern, two special education teachers, one neurolinguist, one speech therapist, one physical therapist, one nurse's aid and two secretaries. Medical specialists from the areas of neurosurgery, neurology, psychiatry and physiatry provide consultation to the program.

Referral is made by the proper authorities concerned with the patient's care, and entrance to the program is decided by the Center's visitation group. Treatment is primarily offered to patients with varied diagnoses (e.g. traumatic brain injury, aneurysm, anoxia, meningoencephalitis, stroke).

Criteria for inclusion in the program are:
1) known etiology of brain damage
2) age 16 years and older
3) good support systems in the family and/or social surroundings
4) possibility of further education or job after completing treatment
5) graduation from primary school ("special education" is acceptable)

6) insight of the patient into his own situation and motivation for treatment. (However, if insight is lacking due to brain damage, a patient will not be excluded).

7) partially preserved ability to communicate

Criteria for exclusion from the program are:

1) the patient is not ambulatory (due to physical limitations at the Center's present location)

2) presence of a progressive CNS illness

3) significant history of substance abuse including alcohol, medicine or drugs

4) long-term psychiatric illness requiring specific treatment

5) presence of chronic deteriorating illnesses.

THE PROGRAM

The main theoretical framework for the program is that of Luria's. Higher cortical processes are conceived of as social in origin, mediated through speech and conscious in their performance. They are considered to be hierarchical, and they are evaluated in accordance with the procedure described in Luria's Neuropsychological Investigation (2). Also the careful qualification of the symptoms that is inherent in the method is stressed with the purpose of gaining insight into the psychological structures and their interrelations. The assessment of each patient according to these principles is strictly individualized. For comparison of outcome with influential Western programs, traditional neuropsychological tests are administered. Furthermore, in order to clarify the emotional and social aspects, assessment of personality and activities of daily life are performed.

The training program is primarily designed in accordance with Luria's model, and consequently built around the resources and disturbances of the individual. The first rule in rehabilitation, according to

Luria, is that patients are fully informed about the
findings of the investigation; awareness of the illness, the situation and the surroundings is considered
a prerequisite for the initiation of training. The
second rule is to make use of brain functions that are
still intact. Thirdly, the training has to be repeated
to the extent of overlearning; the aim being for new
neural pathways to reach automatization. The fourth rule
stresses systematization, the final goal being inter-
nalization of the trained procedures. With the aim of
providing tools for structure and integration, a
specific method has been developed. Continuous written
reviews (made either by patients or therapists, or a
combination thereof) of cognitive and group psychotherapy sessions are collected by the patients and
incorporated into their loose-leaf notebooks.

However, the specific "modular" training described
by Ben Yishay and Diller and their colleagues in the
monographs (3,4) have also had an impact on the development of the program.

Finally, group psychotherapy and individual
therapy has been incorporated as very important addi-
tions to the treatment. The holistic approach as it is
described by Prigatano (5) fits very well with Luria's
concept of the higher cortical processes. The treatment
offered lasts 4 1/2 month, 4 days a week, 6 hours a
day. Ten patients start at the same time and complete
the program together. Each patient is assigned to a
neuropsychologist or a clinical psychologist, who is
responsible for the individual and guides him or her
during the treatment period and afterwards. The goal is
to improve self-awareness and practical abilities,
overcome tendencies toward social withdrawal and to
assist the individual to achieve educational and
professional skills to levels as close as possible to
premorbid functioning.

The activities included in the treatment program are:

1. Morning meeting: The aims are: increase of activity level, concentration and awareness of the environment, orientation to the world, and ability to structure every day life. Activities include review of the day's program and the morning news, as well as, singing and gymnastics. Patients take turns being the leader of the group; their performance is evaluated by group members and therapists.

2. Cognitive Small Group Training: The intent is to improve speed, concentration, orientation, learning, memory, and problem solving. Activities are planned in modules adapted to the patient's needs. Specific methods (e.g. news, television and computer programs) serve as training vehicles.

3. Individual Cognitive Training: Goals are to improve the cognitive and speech disturbances of patients. The activities are planned according to the specific disturbances manifested by the patient. After an initial evaluation, a problem list is developed with associated cognitive remediation tasks. Feedback is given continuously to the patient.

4. Group Psychotherapy: Each therapy session is structured around a specific theme (e.g. reactions to brain damage, changes in personality, relations to family, etc.). Patients take turns discussing each issue. The goals are to enhance motivation, a positive identity and insight into one's strengths and weaknesses as bases for understanding others.

5. Individual Psychotherapy: Support is provided to clarify emotional problems arising throughout the rehabilitation period. Emphasis is placed upon increasing the patient's insight. Additional issues are: making realistic goals, planning the future with regard

to family relations, making good use of free time, and planning future work.

6. Cognitive Social Group: Patients are divided into groups based upon level of functioning and type of social skill problems. Therapy sessions are designed to improve cognitive and social skills through the use of group processes. Games, role playing and imaging (e.g. situations regarding travel, cooking, finances) are a few of the techniques used to improve social skills.

7. Special Education: Individualized special education instruction is provided to improve educational and professional skills. Major academic skills are taught, such as reading, writing, spelling and arithmetic, to levels necessary for a patient to enter into employment or educational programs.

8. Vocal Therapy: In vocal therapy if required the patient is trained to vary the speed, pitch, tempo and volume of speech. Techniques used include: relaxation and training exercises in deep, rhythmic breathing with and without sound. Tonation frequently is used as a training modality. The intent is to compensate for slowed, slurred, often misunderstood speech patterns that cause psychosocial problems.

9. Physiotherapy: Many patients require training to improve body posture, gross and fine motor coordination, balance, respiration, tonus and endurance. Activities include gymnastics, sports (e.g. swimming), massage and training in dressing and personal hygiene. Home visits are made to advise patients about optimal organization and special equipment to compensate for physical disabilities.

10. Relaxation Training: The patient's awareness of a variety of aspects of the body is enhanced through exercise in stretching and coordination of the muscles, autogenic training, visualization and didactic presentations.

11. Vocational Training: In cooperation with employers, with whom the Center has developed collaborative relationships, a patient may have an initial work assignment to test social adaptation and to determine the presence of specific skills necessary to perform a particular job. The assignment precedes work trials supported by the municipalities.

12. Lectures: Weekly lectures are presented by outside specialists on a variety of topics, such as, anatomy and functional organization of the brain, treatment methods, experiences of prior rehabilitation patients, nutrition and interpersonal and sexual relationships.

13. Relatives' Groups: Separate group therapy sessions are held for spouses and for other relatives. Information about brain damage is conveyed. Group members discuss their feelings about living with a brain damaged family member who has personality changes with other individuals in similar situations. Necessary adjustments following improvements during rehabilitation are discussed.

14. Family Consultations: Family members and patient meet with the patient's therapist regularly during the treatment period, discussing emotional and adaptational problems.

15. Family Sessions: Social sessions are held with patients and families, two or three times during the rehabilitation period. The purposes are to acquaint families with the activities at the Center, to meet other patients and relatives and to exchange experiences and hopes.

FOLLOW-UP

After completing the Center's program an intensive follow-up is begun that is an essential part of a successful outcome. Because life crises are more difficult for the brain damaged patient to manage, it is essential that the relationship with the patient's

psychologist can be recreated when required. Only
through the Center's continued long term contacts with
the patient, family and community, is it felt that the
patient will be able to capitalize on the goals reached
during rehabilitation and become reintegrated into
society.

RESEARCH

In order to evaluate the process and the effectiveness of the rehabilitation program of the Center in
relation to different types of head trauma, a controlled clinical study has been developed by a research
committee consisting of professionals involved in the
training program. The evaluation of the rehabilitation
is completed in relation to: neuropsychological,
neurological, activities of daily living, social,
speech and educational level. The study also includes
regional cerebral blood-flow investigations, measured
by Xenon inhalation technique and computed tomography
of the head.

Three patient groups of 25 persons each are
compared: Group 1 consists of patients with traumatic
brain injuries, who receive intensive rehabilitation at
the Center. Group 2 consists of patients with heter-
geneous kinds of brain damage, who receive intensive
rehabilitation at the Center. Group 3 consists of
subjects with the same types of brain damage as Group
1, who receive less intensive treatment elsewhere.(i.e.
mainly physical and occupational therapies without
intensive psychological treatment). Characteristics of
Group 1 and 3 are matched with respect to age, sex,
socioeconomic status, length of time since injury and
depth and length of coma.

Criteria for inclusion in Group 1 are:
1) conformance to the general admission criteria at the
   Center (see above)
2) residence in Sealand or the neighbouring islands

3) occurrence of injury more than one year prior to the start of the program

4) age 16 years and older

5) unconsciousness with the Glasgow Cóma Scale score of eight or less during more than 24 hours.

Criteria for exclusion in Group 1 and 3 include: intracerebral hematoma and skull fractures that require neurosurgical intervention, penetrating lesions of the brain, ventricular hydrocephalus requiring a shunt, malignant or severe physical disorder or incapacities and substance abuse.

The study design implies four evaluations: 1) immediately prior to treatment, 2) immediately after completing treatment period, 3) one-year follow-up and 4) three-year follow-up. For the group of primary interest (Group 1), an evaluation is made six months prior to the onset of treatment. Each evaluation consists of neuropsychological measurements, personality tests and scales, activities of daily living schemas, general personal schemas, physical therapy measurements, communication assessment and cerebral blood flow measurements.

The specific aims of the research program are :

1) the immediate and long-term effects of the Center's rehabilitation program within areas of neuropsychology, emotionality, activities of daily living, and social and economic conditions

2) the outcome comparisons between Groups 1 and 2 of short and long-term rehabilitation.

3) the outcome comparisons between Groups 1 and 3 of short and long-term rehabilitation.

4) the correlatives between the patterns of strengths and deficits observed on neuropsychological examination with disturbances in regional brain-activity and rehabilitation outcomes.

5)   the process of rehabilitation as related to
symptoms and treatment methods.

The research project is an integrated part of the
rehabilitation program, and is considered important
internally, as well as, externally.

REFERENCES

1.   Thomsen, I.V., J.Neurol.Neurosurg.Psychiat.
47:260-268, 1984.
2.   Christensen, A-L., Luria's Neuropsychological
Investigation Text, Munksgaard, Copenhagen, 1984.
3.   Ben-Yishay, Y., Ben-Nachum, Z., Cohen, A., Gross,
Y., Hofien, D., Rattok, J. and Diller, L. Working
Approaches to Remediation of Cognitive Deficits in
Brain Damaged Persons. Institute of Rehabilitation
Medicine, New York University Medical Center, No.
59, New York, 1978.
4.   Ben-Yishay, Y., Working Approaches to Remediation
of Cognitive Deficits in Brain Damaged Persons.
Institute of Rehabilitation Medicine, New York
University Medical Center, No. 63, New York, 1981.
5.   Prigatano, G.P., Fordyce, D.J., Zeiner, H.K.,
Roueche, J.R., Pepping, M. and Wood, B.C. Neuro-
psychological Rehabilitation after Brain Injury,
John Hopkins University Press, Baltimore, 1986.

9

POSTSCRIPT

Barbara P. Uzzell and Anne-Lise Christensen

The complexity of uncontrolled environmental
factors and individual differences of brain damaged
survivors makes a simple approach to successful rehabilitation unlikely. The synergistic efforts of the brain
damaged victim, his family, and many professionals are
required. In this volume, we have advocated a new
approach to rehabilitation based on blending of knowledge of many distinctive fields. We believe this new
wave rehabilitation is more forceful, accelerates
recovery and is beneficial to the brain damaged individual and society.

Because of our beliefs, this book began with
knowledge from a research field devoted to understanding neuromechanisms that underlie behaviors. Easily
incorporated into rehabilitation from this field is the
hypothesis that behavioral changes resulting from
specific goal-directed interventions is accompanied by
plasticity (or the ability of organic systems to
adapt). Such a concept not only provides a basis for
changes following rehabilitation, but a framework to
learn about the plasticity process as well. How the
concept of plasticity is influenced by abruptness and
time of lesion has implications for rehabilitation.
For example, research concerned with plasticity, has
shown that early initiation of rehabilitation following
brain insult insures maximum restoration.

While brain damage results in cellular losses and the breakdown of homeostasis mechanisms, it is also responsible for disruption of neurotransmitter systems within the brain. The situation becomes more complex with the administration of neuropharmacological agents following brain damage, as the effectiveness of these agents will vary with the type of neurotransmitter system that is damaged. Many such agents often affect multiple transmitter systems, so that more than desired change occurs following administration of a neuropharmacological substance. Rehabilitation specialists have just begun to recognize how the interaction between the basic biochemical system of the brain and exdogenous agents influences learning, memory, intellect, and emotional behaviors of brain damaged individuals.

A host of biological and psychological research suggest multidimensional determinants are required in the rehabilitation setting. All aspects of a brain damaged individual's life must be examined. Most particularly, the study of behavioral functioning among the brain damaged, their course of recovery and implications for rehabilitation stress the need to consider the differential pathophysiological events that have impinged upon the nervous system.

The model of rehabilitation for brain damage is different from other forms of rehabilitation. It requires a careful diagnostic system for impairments, environmental content, roles and statuses, self-regulatory functions, executive abilities, and disability acceptance. It requires task analysis interventions appropriately based on careful rehabilitation diagnosis, in order to improve functional competence regardless of whether remediation, re-organization, or compensation skills are taught. It requires the identification of goals and satisfactory assessment of the rehabilitation process. Future directions emphasize in-

tegration of knowledge outside the field of rehabilitation and long-term restorative aspects.

While advances in brain-injured treatment and
rehabilitation management are extensive and costly,
appropriate treatment has been shown to lessen prospec-
tive costs. Benefits of new wave rehabilitation have
been cost-effective. Those involved in financial
aspects, whether they represent state programs or
private insurance sources have begun to understand the
individual's rehabilitation requirements and have
encouraged accountability of the rehabilitation facilities.

The discussions from the chapters of this book
indicate that the model for new wave rehabilitation
comes from education and psychology, not medicine.
Recent outcome studies of brain damaged individuals
show the main problems are psychological and social. It
is our contention that the integration of knowledge
from various disciplines into the rehabilitation
process will assist in minimizing these main problems.
In order to do this, rehabilitation specialists need to
plan for a full course of treatment using accumulated
knowledge of various fields, and to recognize differences among individuals in spontaneous recovery, and
their cognitive and emotional growth. The possibilities
for socializing need to be carried out in a structured
manner, so that the brain damaged survivor will not
have to live a restricted life.

We hope in some small way this book will contribute to the ultimate rehabilitation goal of promoting improved quality of life for brain damaged individuals.

INDEX

Activities of daily living (ADL)
  assessment of, 72, 74
  disabilities and, 61, 64
  rehabilitation programs with, 54
Acute care programs, 57
Affective disorder, neuropharmacology
    for, 25
Agitation, neuropharmacology for, 26–27,
    31, 35
Alcoholic induced dementia, 26
Alzheimer's dementia, 26
American Psychiatric Association, 21
Amnesia Association (Amnass), 80–81
Amnesia, post-traumatic, 30
Amphetamine
  attention deficit disorders (ADD) and, 31
  cognitive deficits treatment with, 26
  comatose or poorly aroused patient and,
    25
  hemiplegia treatment with, 22
  traumatic head injury and, 35
Anticholinesterase agents, and memory
    function, 26
Anticonvulsant medications, 33–35
Anti-depressant medications, 35
  attention deficit disorders (ADD) and,
    30–31
  seizures and, 29
Antipsychotic medications, 35
  anticholinergic action of, 29–30
  long-term use of, 30
  tardive dyskinesia and, 21
  traumatic brain damage (TBI) and, 29
Antispasticity agents, 32
Aphasia
  haloperidol treatment of, 22
  rehabilitation for, 82–84
  time factors in recovery from, 13
Assessment
  behavioral techniques in, 73–74
  categories of behavior in, 74–76
  commonly used procedures in, 70–71
  criticism of, 72–73
  early procedures for, 70–76
  quality of life issues in, 63
  neuropsychological, 111–112

rehabilitation and, 60–61
research on, 74–76
stimulation and, 77
Attention deficit disorders (ADD),
    neuropharmacology for, 30–31
Attention disorders, neuropsychological
    rehabilitation for, 44–45, 47–49
Auditory stimulation procedures, 76

Baker, E., 83
Barnes, R., 29
Barthel Scale, 72
Basso, A., 42
Behavioral approaches
  assessment and, 73–74
  rehabilitation and, 78–79
Behavioral deficits
  serial lesions and, 5–6
  variables affecting degree of, 8
Ben-Yishay, Y., 65, 66, 118
Benzodiazepines, 31–32
Bereweeke programme, 74
Berry, T., 83
Beta-blocker medications, 35
Bieliauskas, L.A., 44
Biering-Sørensen, Fin, 104, 107
Bipolar disease, 32
Bistany, Diane V., 87–101
Boyle, M.E., 77
Brain
  definition of plasticity and, 2–4
  types of realities about organization of,
    1–2, 16
Brain damage
  contextual factors in recovery from, 4–8
  depressive phenomena in, 25
  design of a rehabilitation program and
    type of, 70
  localizationist perspective on, 6
  neuronal sprouting in response to, 14–15
  neuropsychological rehabilitation of, 39–52
  recovery from, see Recovery from brain
    damage
  serial lesions and, 4–6
  see also Traumatic brain damage (TBI)